i

INTRODUCTION

This text is designed to provide a complete, yet concise review of the
available literature regarding the science and practice of hydrotherapy.
This publication is not intended to replace qualified medical care. The author and
publisher accept no responsibility for the use of the information contained herein by its
readers. If questions regarding the appropriateness of any treatment should arise, a
qualified medical practitioner should be consulted.

3rd Edition – 2003   ISBN 097119261-8   Pine Island Publishers Inc.

2nd Edition 1997
1st Edition 1995

For information on this and other publications please contact:

Pine Island Publishers Inc.   **Websites: www.PineIslandPublishers.com**
Phone: 1-800-400-1892   **www.examreviews.com**

PREFACE

"Modern scientific research has placed upon a sure foundation the great truth - dimly recognized by the earliest physicians, but wholly lost sight of during the dark ages - that healing power is not possessed by physicians nor by remedies, but that the curative process is simply a manifestation of the forces which dwell within the body and which are normally manifested in creating and maintaining the organism; in other words, the body heals itself. Water, applied externally or internally, and at such temperatures as may be required, is an agent which more fully than almost any other cooperates with the healing powers of the body in resisting the onset and development of pathogenic processes. There is no other remedy by which the movements of the blood and the blood supply, both general and local, and in fact every form of vital activity, may be so readily controlled as by hydriatic applications."

The above quote is from the preface of *Rational Hydrotherapy* and was written by Dr. John Harvey Kellogg in 1899. These words penned by the famous doctor nearly one hundred years ago are still true as we enter the 21st Century. Although the popular fervor for hydrotherapy during the late 19th and early 20th Centuries has waned, the value of this therapeutic tool remains great. This book has been written with the hope that the science and practice of hydrotherapy will grow and prosper in the coming millennium. The author intends that his interest and respect for this modality might be contagious to those who read this text.

This text is intended to be a resource for both education and clinical practice. Contained herein are sections regarding the history, philosophy, and principles of hydrotherapy, along with a brief discussion of pertinent anatomical and physiological data. Numerous therapeutic and spa techniques are described in detail, as well as guidelines for their use. A brief discussion of fever, as it applies to hydrotherapy, is also included. Lastly, the reader will find a section describing several forms of heliotherapy, an allied modality.

The author and co-contributors have made an earnest effort to exclude from this work any information, which is without scientific and physiological foundation. Knowing that this work will not be found without fault, we solicit the candid criticism of those who would pay us the honor of reading these pages, trusting that the author will have the privilege of correcting in future editions any errors as may have escaped his attention and to record such new facts as future research and knowledge may reveal.

ACKNOWLEDGMENTS

The author wishes to extend his deepest appreciation to all those who have played a part in bringing this text to fruition: I especially thank Leigh Reynolds, L.Ac. for her technical contributions and personal support. Kay Hugghins, J.D. is greatly appreciated for her final editing of the entire text. My gratitude goes to Christine Heffner for her contributions to the Anatomy & Physiology and Hydrotherapy Techniques sections. James Megonnell was an invaluable source of technical guidance during production. Recognition must go to Dr. David Epley, Jean Reese, Isabelle Dunkeson and all my students for allowing me to teach. To my mother who encouraged me to read, to question, and to think, I am forever grateful.

ABOUT THE AUTHOR

Dr. Patrick Barron received both his Bachelor's and Master's Degrees in Rehabilitation from Marshall University. His Doctorate in Naturopathic Medicine was earned from Bastyr University. He completed two years Post Doctoral training at the University of Washington and has been in private practice specializing in Rehabilitation Medicine for over 19 years. Dr. Barron is the director of Oviedo Physical Medicine, a medical and educational consulting group. He is the founder of the Central Florida School of Health Sciences and is currently Professor of Clinical Medicine at the Florida College of Integrative Medicine in Orlando.

TABLE OF CONTENTS

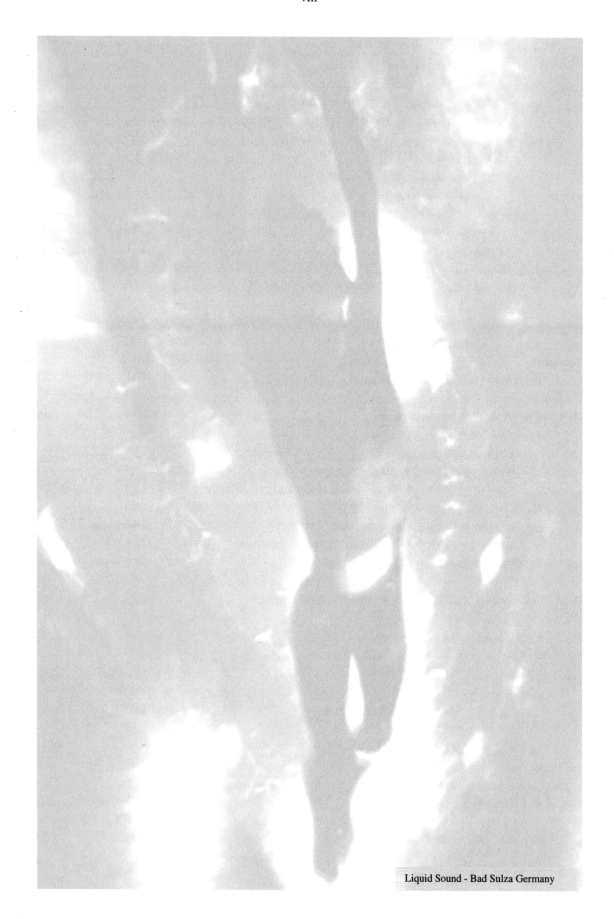

Liquid Sound - Bad Sulza Germany

I. HISTORY OF HYDROTHERAPY

Ancient Hydrotherapy (? - 1299 A.D.)

The history of hydrotherapy has been influenced by overlapping and diversely opposing points of view -- orthodox medical doctors, unorthodox medical practitioners, native healers, and believers who learned through experience. The use of hydrotherapy is documented in the western world as far back as the Greek and Roman Era. Chinese and Japanese records from several centuries B.C. record prescriptions of cold water affusions. The Japanese used bathing, especially outdoor baths, for meditation and maintaining balance with the forces of nature. For centuries, bathing in wooden tubs of hot water has been a Japanese ritual. Ancient Egyptians, Hebrews, Persians, and Hindus all used water in the treatment of disease, as do their descendants today. Native Americans inhabited areas near hot mineral springs for thousands of years before Europeans came to America. The ancient tradition of sweat bathing continues today among many tribal cultures.

 Some of the earliest records of mankind refer to "wash and be healed." People instinctively used water when sick, one of the earliest forms of the healing arts. The Bible refers to the daughter of Pharaoh and her attendants going down to the Nile. Homer speaks of the bathing habits of his heroes. The Old and New Testaments mention bathing as a cleansing and healing process, as well as a religious rite. Ancient Jews regarded bathing as an ascetic activity and the bath was used for cleansing only. However, later contact with the Babylonians introduced the Jews to Sumerian bathing practices. Bathing was then viewed as necessary for spiritual purification, as well as for physical cleanliness. Throughout early medical history and up until the early 20th Century, many distinguished physicians and medical writings recommended the remedial use of water in the treatment of diseases such as measles, typhoid fever, dyspepsia (digestive disorders), gout, rheumatism, scarlatina, and erysipelas (contagious skin infection). Many surgeons of this era and of earlier times thought that water was a preferable dressing (over cataplasms, poultices, and liniments) for wounds, swelling, and inflammation.

Ancient baths were considered spiritual, hygienic, therapeutic and social. According to Siegfried Giedion's *Mechanization Takes Command*, "The role that bathing plays within a culture reveals the culture's attitude toward human relaxation. It is a measure of how far individual well-being is regarded as an indispensable part of community life."

The Greeks favored cleanliness but bathing was not an indulgence. They bathed after strenuous workouts and prior to intellectual discussions at gymnasiums. The gymnasium was the educational core of their society, and the therapeutic use of water was an essential part of the institution. Ruins of baths built between 1700 and 1400 B.C. have been found in Crete. The Spartans felt so strongly about bathing, they made it mandatory by law.

Hippocrates (460-377 B.C.)
The "Father of Medicine," prescribed the use of cold bath and friction in the treatment of both acute and chronic disease. Records indicate that water was used in treating fever, inflammation, gout, and rheumatism, as well as many other illnesses. Because of the calming effects of water, it was also used in treating the mentally disturbed. Aristotle, who was a student of Plato, opened the first western university in Athens in the year 347 B.C. and hygiene was included as a part of the curriculum. The Greeks first used only cold baths. Later documents report the use of hot water and steam bathing as well as the use of sponges, oils, rinses, and a metal instrument called a strigil for scraping oneself to collect what was eliminated by the pores.

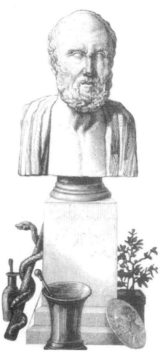

Hippocrates of Cos

The Romans took the bath to new heights. Bathing was ritualized and became an art form. A Roman poet coined the phrase *"mens sana in corpore sano"* (a sound mind in a sound body). Romans believed in equilibrium for wholeness and created environments for maintaining that equilibrium. The earliest known Roman baths are the Stabian baths built in the 2nd century B.C. at Pompeii. Their design is similar to others found throughout the empire. The Roman *thermae* (baths) were institutions that reflected a holistic conception of health. Roman baths were created for health and treating disease, but evolved into a social occasion as well. For centuries, separate baths were used by men and women, with women's baths being smaller versions of the elaborate originals. Toward the end of the Roman Empire, men and women bathed together and the baths became associated with debauchery. About 138 A.D., the current ruler prohibited mixed bathing. Changes in the use of the baths were made to once again accommodate separate bathing and regulate the use of the baths. The Romans used physical therapy, as well as hydrotherapy, for treatment. The famous Roman physician Celsus, who wrote an encyclopedia of medicine, later added the modalities of exercise and massage to his therapeutic system. Few houses had private baths. The public baths were attractive and a very interesting meeting place. Public bathing was so popular that five imperial *thermae* were built in Rome between the 1st and 4th Centuries A.D. The extensive ruins of three of these baths remain. Water was piped in from the town's aqueduct; the furnace room contained pipes, boiler, and a wood supply. The floors and walls, which were made of mosaic tile were heated by a hypocaust which circulated heated air through a system of flues. The bathhouse consisted of an *apodyterium* (dressing room), a *frigidarium* (cold bath), a *tepidarium* (tepid bath), a *caldarium* (hot bath), and possibly a *palaestra* (exercise court). More elaborate baths might also include a *laconium* (room of intense dry heat similar to the Finnish sauna). The routine often included a turn in the warm room (tepidarium) or the hot room (caldarium--which might include a hot water immersion tank), depending on their preference. From these rooms, the bathers plunged into the cold water room (frigidarium). After these treatments, they would receive a massage and relax in the garden with their friends. Some baths included libraries, ornate decorations, arcades, garden paths, fountains, and music for soothing the nerves. The bath experience was considered to be invigorating, cleansing, and restorative.

 To both the Romans and Greeks, the body was an object of admiration and they kept it clean -- unlike many western European cultures, which were indifferent to filth. As the power and influence of classic Rome declined, and partially because of the early Christian rejection or denial of the body, both public and private bathing were discouraged.
Bathing, particularly in chilly northern Europe, came to be viewed as unhealthy and was frowned upon as an unnecessary indulgence. Dirt was a badge of holiness and not washing oneself was considered a pious act of self-denial. Medieval city planners were more concerned with fortification than with water supply and drainage. Most of Europe suffered from a complete disorganization and disruption of medical care. By the Fifth Century A.D., Europe had forgotten the bathing practices of the Romans and Greeks. Cleanliness reached an all-time low from the Sixteenth to Nineteenth Century. People used perfumes and cosmetics as a substitute for bathing. Although many late medieval communities had public baths, offering both refreshment and entertainment, these facilities were considered to be quite disreputable. Bathing among Europeans was rare, with only the Jews retaining a concept of cleanliness during this period. Their religion required them to take frequent baths. *The Name of the Rose* starring Sean Connery is a relatively current film giving much insight into the prevalent attitude of most Europeans during this period (and previously) toward the study of health, hygiene, and science in general. Intellectual stagnation, superstition, and fear were the norm for most of Europe during medieval times. Folklore and magic replaced science and knowledge. Books were destroyed, while midwives and herbalists burned at the stake, accused as heretics and witches. Even in the great cities such as Constantinople, a series of epidemics served to strengthen the belief that disease was caused by evil. Medicine in general, and certainly not the use of a natural element such as water had any place in the treatment of disease, which was considered to be a purely spiritual concern. Only in the monasteries of Europe did knowledge persist, as monks continued the laborious task of collecting, studying, and duplicating by hand the classic medical texts.

 During the Middle (Dark) Ages, Arabic physicians preserved the classic Greek and Roman tradition and continued to advocate the use of hydrotherapy. The Islamic countries became the main repository of classic western scientific thought. The great library at Alexandria, which was founded by Ptolemy I, King of Egypt (4th Century B.C.) contained over 40,000 books. As legend holds, the library was sacked and burned on three separate occasions by Christian Roman Emperors. It is largely through the survival of the classic texts held in the Arabic world that we have today the knowledge of Hippocrates, Celsus, and others. Not only did water have a therapeutic and hygienic use, but the Muslims believed that relaxed bathing led to enlightenment. Rejuvenation was a spiritual issue, and the bath or *hamam* became the Islamic water temple. At the height of bathing, Baghdad had over 30,000 bathhouses. The ritual of bathing continues today in the Muslim countries, with facilities being available to both men and women.

In northeastern Europe, where Roman influence was minimal and the Catholic Church took longer to become established, the Finns and Russians developed a spiritual, as well as social attitude toward bathing. The *Sauna* developed from the ancient steam baths of the Scythian nomads. Finnish and Russian families built small wooden rooms or huts with benches. Water was thrown on heated stones to produce clouds of steam in which the bathers sweated. They soaped, rubbed, and flogged themselves with birch twigs, ending the ritual with a plunge into icy water or snow. The sauna was often the first building to be constructed when starting a family after marriage. The sauna was a place of healing. Babies were born in saunas, and the dead were laid out in them before funerals.

Modern Hydrotherapy (1300 A.D. to Present)

The repressive and unenlightened views of medieval society were beginning to wane towards the latter portion of the Dark Ages. St. Thomas Aquinas (circa 1300 A.D.) wrote and spoke of the virtues of cleanliness. He was no doubt influenced by the classic Greek and Roman literature, which had been preserved in the Arabic world, as some of his writings bear great similarities to the Greek masters. John Wesley, founder of Methodism, recognized therapeutic public bathing in the eighteenth century and he preached, "cleanliness is next to godliness." He believed that cold baths could cure some fifty afflictions. He extolled the virtues of cold water in the treatment of fever in his book *Primitive Physick*. Vapor baths became very popular in the Seventeenth and Eighteenth Centuries in France. Barbers were considered men of medicine and frequently used hydrotherapy treatments. Lack of plumbing during the industrial revolution made hygiene impossible (yet even more needed). Lack of cleanliness contributed to the severity of the cholera epidemic in 1832 and subsequent outbreaks. Fifty thousand people died. As a result, the British were motivated to develop indoor plumbing.

Forbes of London was the physician to Queen Victoria and practiced hydrotherapy. John Floyer (1649-1734) wrote a book, *The History of Hot and Cold Bathing*, which went into six editions. He influenced a great number of people. His book was translated into German in 1749 and influenced Dr. Johann Sigmund Hahn (1696-1773), who then established the principles of modern hydrotherapy in Germany.

Vincent Priessnitz (1799-1852), an Austrian, had great success with water treatments. He had no formal education, but was recognized because of his successful treatments. He was persecuted by the medical authorities of his day and convicted of using witchcraft because he taught people to heal themselves by the use of water, air, diet, and exercise. He was described by Dr. John Kellogg as an "uneducated, blundering peasant that brought the world's attention to the use of hydrotherapy." Priessnitz was however, one of the first Europeans to carefully organize and document the effects of water in its various modes of application. In spite of his persecution, many medical doctors traveled to his home to learn these treatments because of the success he experienced with his patients. Priessnitz influenced many people involved in the development and use of hydrotherapy.

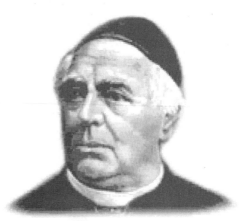

Father Sebastian Kneipp

The most influential individual following Priessnitz was **Father Sebastian Kneipp** (1821-1897). Kneipp was stricken with tuberculosis at age 25 and cured himself with water and diet therapies after reading a pamphlet written by Dr. Johann Sigmund Hahn. Kneipp's book, *My Water Cure*, published in 1886, greatly influenced the development of hydrotherapy in the United States. Kneipp taught of the five pillars of health; hydrotherapy, herbal therapy, diet therapy, kinesiotherapy, and lifestyle management. His patients included imperial and royal families, such as the Prince of Wales, King Edward VIII, Baron Rothschild, Pope Leo XIII, and other high dignitaries in the Church. He never charged for his services. In 1891, Father Kneipp treated Benedict Lust and cured his medical problems. Lust was restored to good health through the teachings of water, air, food, herbs, earth, and sunshine. Kneipp's teachings became the corner stone of the "Nature Cure" movement. Lust later brought Kneipp's teachings and methods to America and influenced Dr. John Harvey Kellogg and **Frederick W. Collins**, M.D., D.O., N.D., D.C., A.M., pioneer hydropathist and author of *The Simplicity of the Water Cure.* His hydrotherapy treatments included: hot water packs, compresses, ablutions of the entire body, health baths, steam baths, enemas, baths for affected body parts, fever reducing packs, cold packs, sitz baths, and rubbing methods. Father Kneipp's treatments were extensive; some are listed and include: abdominal spasm, arthritis, rheumatism, asthma, bladder infections and stones, bleeding, inflammations, cancer (the aim was to rid the body of impurities and maintain the general strength of the patient), cholera, delirium, diabetes mellitus, dislocations and sprains, drunkenness, cataracts, fever, gastric complaints, headaches, heart disease, hip-joint inflammation, hysteria, insomnia, lumbago, lupus, mental diseases, migraines, atrophy of the muscles (unhealthy changes in the nervous system affect the supply of blood and ultimately the health of the muscle - treatment was to improve circulation), affections of the nerves, nervousness, paralysis, sciatica, spinal complaints, stiff neck, syphilis, varicose veins, wounds, and writer's cramp. Bathing had two purposes; to cleanse the body of impurities and perspiration, and to refresh the body and soul. Packs and compresses were commonly used to treat inflammation and purify the blood.

Hydrotherapy first became prominent in America during the 1840s. Henry Wadsworth Longfellow and Harriet Beecher Stowe were prominent patrons of the Brattleboro Infirmary in Vermont. The *Water Cure Journal* published by Joel Shew (1816-1855), had a circulation of about 50,000 copies. He was an invalid and was purportedly cured of overexposure to mercury, iodine, and bromine compounds with which he worked.

One of Shew's associates, Russell Thatcher Trall (1812-1877), established a water-cure house in New York City. He wrote *The Hydropathic Encyclopedia* and established the Hygieo-Therapeutic College in New York City, which included instruction in medicine, electricity, Swedish movement, gymnastics, diet, and water treatment. He attempted to separate himself from the more radical hydropathists who claimed all diseases could be cured by cold water alone. J.H. Pulte (1811-1884) and H. P. Gatchell (1815-1889), two prominent homeopaths, published the <u>*American Magazine of Homeopathy and Hydropathy*</u> in the Mid-19th Century. Mary Gove Nichols (1810-1884), a women's rights and health reformer, and her husband, Thomas Low Nichols, founded the American Hydropathic Institute in New York; a coeducational medical school, based on water cure principles.

The popularity of hydropathy began to decline in the late 19th Century. However, James Caleb Jackson treated thousands of patients in his "home of the hillside" in Dansville, New York. He claimed a 95% success rate. He believed his treatments were most effective when combined with other hygienic measures; nutrition, fresh air, exercise, dress, sleep, etc. One of his articles introduced **Ellen G. White** (1827-1915), the founder of Seventh Day Adventism and health reformer, to hydrotherapy. She was very concerned with the continuing use of "poisonous drugs" by the current medical profession. The use of arsenic and mercury (in the treatment of syphilis) were common practices, as well as that of blood letting. She later sponsored the work of Dr. John Harvey Kellogg, one of the most important figures in the modern history of hydrotherapy.

Dr. John Harvey Kellogg (1852-1943), helped establish and run the famous Battle Creek Sanitarium in Michigan. His 1,260-page work *Rational Hydrotherapy* appeared in 1901 and still remains the definitive textbook on hydrotherapy. His sanitarium was very popular. Affluent people from all over the world came to this sanitarium for treatment. The sanitarium used advanced diet therapy, hydrotherapy and massage, as well as current medical procedures. Most treatments included non-drug and surgical procedures as well as physiotherapeutic modalities. Dr. Kellogg was considered by many to be the greatest physician of his time. He was known worldwide for his use of hydrotherapy and his inventive genius.

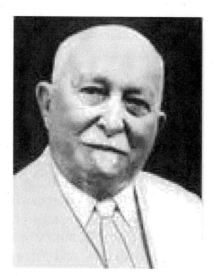

John Harvey Kellogg, MD

He is credited with developing corn flakes, peanut butter, the electric blanket, and other electrotherapy devices. He treated serious infections, pneumonia, pyelonephritis, and post-operative and pre-operative pain with hydrotherapy. Dr. Kellogg was also known for his overbearing nature and extreme views regarding colon hygiene and chastity. The 1994 film *The Road to Wellville* portrays Dr. Kellogg (played by Anthony Hopkins), in a somewhat unflattering, yet no doubt accurate fashion.

Simon Baruch (1840-1921) attempted to separate water treatments from the unschooled believers and establish it as part of orthodox medicine. His works, *The Principles and Practices of Hydrotherapy* (1898) and *An Epitome of Hydrotherapy* (1920) are valuable, but failed to convert the mainstream medical society.

Henry Lindlahr (1852-1925) was a real estate tycoon, mayor, banker, and leading citizen of Kalispell, Montana. At age 41 he found out he had diabetes mellitus. After being told by the best American doctors that his time was limited, he went to Europe. He visited Father Kneipp. After Father Kneipp's initial observations, he was told to take sitz baths, live on fruits, greens and vegetables, and avoid all sugar, breads, cereals, and meats. After being healed, he returned to the United States and studied medicine and established a sanitarium in Chicago. The basement of his sanitarium utilized extensive hydrotherapeutic equipment. He wrote a book, *Nature Cure*, which was read by anyone who wanted to practice hydrotherapy.

Dr. O.G. Carroll (1879-1962) developed a constitutional hydrotherapy treatment. As a child, he suffered rheumatic fever and juvenile arthritis. He studied under Lindlahr. He moved to Spokane, Washington and became one of the first naturopathic practitioners in the West. He established a sanitarium in Spokane, which ran until his death in 1962. He was a fearless practitioner. It is said, that he cured Dr. Kellogg's wife of asthma.

Dr. John Bastyr, one of that eras greatest physicians, studied with Dr. Carroll and continued to integrate his own version of the constitutional treatment with other natural therapies. Dr. Bastyr treated patients at his office in Seattle until a short time before his death in 1995. Dr. Harold Dick of Spokane, Washington, was a renowned hydrotherapist. After seeing the success of Dr. Carroll's treatments on his brother, Dr. Dick was formally trained by Drs. Carroll and Bastyr. **Dr. A.C. Johnson**, a Chiropractor and Naturopath published the notable *Principles and Practice of Drugless Therapeutics* in 1965.

As late as 1927, hydrotherapy was still a mainstream method of treatment in the United States. The American Medical Association recognized the powerful effects water had in treating disease. Neutral or tepid baths, used for a long period of time, were effective in treating excited mental cases. The Brand Bath was used to treat typhoid fever, stimulating the nervous system, the circulatory system, and the immune system. The cold friction mitt was used to treat some cases of bronchopneumonia in young patients. Also, acute infections, as well as chronic diseases and rehabilitation, were treated by hydrotherapy. The *Journal of American Medical Association* reported in 1936 that hydrotherapy was useful for Sydenham's chorea, gonorrhea, and other conditions.

Of all the contributors discussed, Priessnitz and Kneipp's works remain the basis for modern hydrotherapy. Dr. Kellogg put hydrotherapy on a scientific footing. Lust and Lindlahr, pioneers in naturopathy, incorporated hydrotherapy in their teachings and practices. Drs. Carroll, Bastyr, Johnson, and Dick were the most prominent recent contributors. Dr. Dick is quoted as saying, "Our job is to make over the blood. Until we do, we're just spinning our wheels."

The popularity and practice of hydrotherapy, as well as many other natural remedies, continued to decline after the early 20th Century. This decline continued because hydrotherapy treatments take longer to apply and monitor, and their effects are generally much slower and less dramatic than those delivered by drug therapy. Many treatments are just as effective as drug therapy and do not have the side effects--however; they require time and skill on the part of the therapist, and understanding on the part of the patient. The public, as well as the medical profession, no longer remember when the proper use of hydrotherapy, exercise, diet control, and massage were used to treat illnesses such as pneumonia, rheumatic fever, typhoid, and polio before the discovery of antibiotics. Medical schools have long disagreed over the best methods of treatment. As a result, medical schools branched into various schools of teaching: allopathy, homeopathy, osteopathy, chiropractic, naturopathy, and others. For most of the past 50 years, the tenets of practical hydrotherapy have been nurtured by a few chiropractic and naturopathic physicians, 7th Day Adventist practitioners, physical therapists, and massage therapists.

Development of Spas

Spa is defined as a resort known for its baths and mineral springs. Spa, a town in eastern Belgium in Liege Province was frequented in Roman times and later in the 18th and 19th Centuries. It was a fashionable resort visited by royalty. The name of the town, Spa, later became the generic name given to mineral baths. Early spas were simply wells, pools, or mineral springs thought to have healing abilities-- spiritual as well as physical cures. How they healed was a mystery. Many thought that it was not the water, but the forces in the water, that cured. Both Perrier, in the south of France and Ferralelle, in southern Italy, claim that Hannibal and his armies used their spas. There were three main types of water. Saline waters contained dissolved salts or magnesium sulfate used primarily for its purgative effects; chalybeate waters

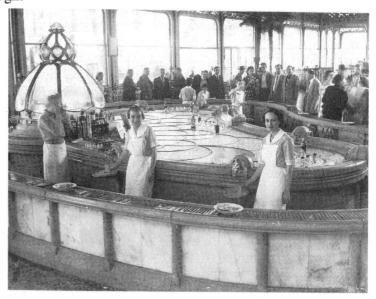

Water Bar at Vichy, France - Circa 1925

turned rust-colored when the ferrous carbonate (iron) was exposed to air and were used primarily for tonic and restorative effects, and sulfur waters contained hydrogen sulfide and were used primarily for bathing, drinking, and to treat the skin. These natural spas also varied in temperature and degree of natural effervescence.

The Reformation changed the ideas of how water healed. The water was no longer credited with mystical powers and doctors came into the picture. Cleanliness improved general health conditions. Spas actually became hospitals during this time. In France, as well as most other European countries, *thermalisme* (thermal healing) was taken very seriously and actually taught as a course in medical schools. Drinking waters high in mineral content were recommended to cure everything from kidney stones to heart conditions. The overindulgent wealthy recognized the healing capacity of these waters and demanded accommodations that fit their lifestyle. By the middle of the nineteenth century, spas reflected the wealthy tastes of their clientele. From Roman time until the 1930s, the list of visitors included: Julius Caesar, Michelangelo, Montaigne, Casanova, Napoleon and Josephine, Queen Victoria, Victor Hugo, Tolstoy, Henry James, Charles Dickens, William Makepeace Thackeray, Jane Austen, Chopin, and Agatha Christie to name a few. England, France, Germany, Belgium, Italy, Switzerland, and Czechoslovakia built famous and luxurious spas during this time. With the decline of the upper class and the two world wars, spa popularity declined. However, spa culture experienced a revival in the mid 1980s. Bill Keysing, in his *Great Hot springs of the West* (1984) stated: "It may well be that water extracts a subtle energy from deep within the earth and transmits it to truthseekers. Or perhaps the relaxation of the body, while immersed in soothing warm water, creates a new and enlightened ecology of the mind, allowing quantum leaps in understanding".

American spas developed as natural hot springs were discovered. Native Americans long recognized the special cures that hot springs had to offer. People went to the spas seeking relaxation of the body and soul. Hot spring resorts popped up. Their popularity declined after the 1930s because of the World War I and the competition of new vacation spots. The therapeutic reputation of mineral waters suffered a decline with the drug industry's production of artificial healing agents (and societies desire for a quick cure). However, in the 1960s, health enthusiasts, environmentalists, and spiritualists again rediscovered the magic of hot springs that Saratoga Springs in New York, Hot Springs in Arkansas, Safety Harbor in Florida, and White Sulphur Springs in West Virginia have persevered. Modern spas pamper the mind as well as the body -- balancing the left and right sides of the brain, biofeedback, mind healing, life-style changes, Tai Chi, yoga, meditation, breathing, massage and visualization are methods used to reduce stress, and a healthy diet is provided along with exercise to help maintain a healthy body. Traditional spas include Saratoga Springs in New York, Calistoga in California, Boyes Hot Springs and Sonoma Mission Inn in California, and Two Bunch Palms in Desert Hot Springs, California. Super spas of today include Rancho La Puerta in Baja California, Golden Door in Escondido, California, and Cal-a-Vie in Vista, California. Modern spas utilize massage and other relaxation techniques, as well as hydrotherapy techniques including whirlpools, sauna baths, Russian baths, salt glows, peloids (mineral mud) and fango (moor peat) baths, and mineral water baths. Alev L. Croutier, author of *Taking the Waters*, compares European and American spas and states, "European spas are filled with history and the spirit of gifted people whose art, music or philosophy were admired. They are romantic and nostalgic. American spas are unsurpassed in their level of pampering. Each are very expensive". The French physician Deslois-Paoli was asked why spa cures work. He replied, "We really don't know. There are two reasons. One is the effect of the waters themselves; the other is admittedly the psychosomatic effect." This is not unlike many modern medical treatments, which work, but the mechanisms remain unexplained.

Over thousands of years, the therapeutic use of water has been studied, developed, and recorded. Ancient cultures established rituals, which persist even into the 20th century. Early scientists such as Hippocrates and Celsius have bestowed upon us knowledge, which appears to be timeless. Their information survived the medieval period due largely to preservation in the monasteries of Europe and in libraries of the Arabic world. Modern era pioneers like Priessnitz, Kneipp, and Kellogg have contributed much towards our understanding of hydrotherapy. To these and others that remain unnamed, we are indebted.

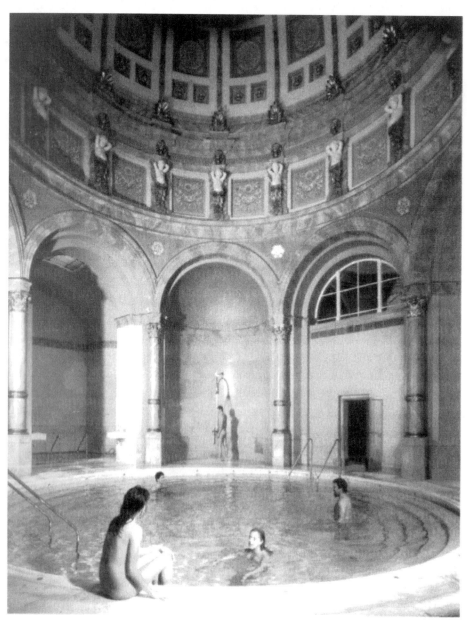

Roman-Irish Bathhouse at Baden-Baden, Germany - Built Circa 1880

CHAPTER I SUMMARY - HISTORY OF HYDROTHERAPY:

(dates below are approximate)

2000 BC,   Chinese, Hindu, Egyptian & Hebrew cultures begin to write about the therapeutic use of bathing.

1700 BC,   Sumerians, Cretans, Babylonians build elaborate baths.

460-377 BC, Hippocrates (aka: **Father of Modern Medicine**) teaches about herbs, diet, exercise and hydrotherapy.

400 BC,   Library at Alexandria built by King Ptolemy I.

200 BC,   First of many Roman baths built at Pompeii.

400 AD,   Decline of the Roman Empire and beginning of the Dark Ages.

1300 AD,   St. Thomas Aquinas writes about the virtues of cleanliness.

1700 AD,   John Wesley (founder of Methodism) extols the virtues of hydrotherapy in his book *The Primitive Physick*.

1730 AD,   John Floyer writes *The History of Hot & Cold Bathing*.

1830 AD,   Vincent Priessnitz (aka: **Founder of Modern Hydrotherapy**) organizes & documents hydrotherapy practices of the day.

1850 AD,   Joel Shew publishes the *Water Cure Journal* with a circulation of over 50,000.

1880 AD,   Ellen White (founder of 7th Day Adventism and noted health reformer) sponsors the work of Dr. John Harvey Kellogg.

1886 AD,   Fr. Sebastian Kneipp (aka: **Father of Modern Hydrotherapy**) develops his theories of health care and writes *My Water Cure*.

1898 AD,   Simon Baruch writes *The Principles and Practices of Hydrotherapy*.

1901 AD,   Dr. John Harvey Kellogg treats thousands of patients at his Battle Creek Sanitarium and writes his 1,260 page *Rational Hydrotherapy*.

1925 AD,   Henry Lindlahr writes *Nature Cure.*

1965 AD,   Dr. A.C. Johnson, Chiropractor and Naturopath writes the notable *Principles and Practice of Drugless Therapeutics.*

1984 AD,   Wm. Keysing writes *Great Hot Springs of the West.*

1980's
to date: Rebirth of the American spa.

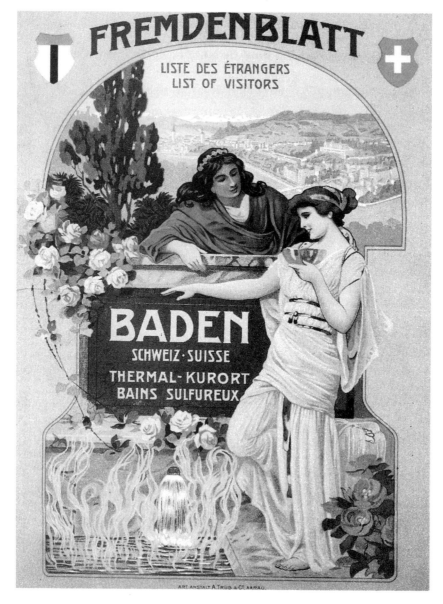

Spa Poster from Baden, Switzerland - Circa 1900

II. THEORY OF HYDROTHERAPY

A. Introduction

In order to prevent any misunderstandings, the more commonly used descriptive terms in hydrotherapy and their definitions are listed in the glossary. Hydrotherapy is defined as the application of water in its three forms (solid, liquid, or vapor) to the body, either externally or internally, in the treatment of disease or trauma. These methods include but are not limited to: sitz bath, douche, spa and hot tub, whirlpool, sauna, shower, immersion bath, pack, poultice, foot bath, fomentation, and wrap. "Internal use" typically refers to drinking mineral waters, using irrigations, or administering enemas and colonic irrigations. It is understood that the practice of hydrotherapy may also include the use of herbal and chemical preparations applied in conjunction with applications of water -- such as with the use of plasters, poultices masks, wraps, and baths.

Most commonly, therapists focus on the external use of hot and cold. Understanding why a technique is used and the individual needs of each client/patient is most important and can enhance the treatment. There are variables affecting each treatment. The therapist can control the temperature, duration, and extent of each treatment, but not the disease/condition, vitality of the client/patient or his/her tolerance for the treatment. In as much as hydrotherapy is a powerful tool, it may also produce unwanted results if not used in a conscientious and scientific manner.

Knowledge of certain physical and physiological principles is necessary for an effective hydrotherapy treatment-- water has certain properties; the temperature has local and general effects upon the body; and different methods of application have different effects. Homeostasis is the term used to describe the optimum stable condition of the healthy human body-- the body continually initiates physiological processes in an attempt to maintain the stability of its internal environment in response to external changes. These physiological changes are usually in direct proportion to the extent of external changes. Hydrotherapy changes the environment of the body by the application of water at varying temperatures.

B. Philosophy of Hydrotherapy

Health and healing are proportional to the normal flow of healthy blood--the quantity and quality of the blood flowing to the tissue. Hydrotherapy's goal is to normalize the quantity of blood circulating through a given area during a given period of time by manipulating its circulation. Its purpose is to excite the vital force or "Vis Medicatrix Naturae" by means of methodical thermic applications. For certain situations this would mean an increase in circulation, while in others it would be a decrease; i.e. hot water will help relax a tight muscle or an ice pack can limit the swelling of a sprained ankle. In other words, it is not the power of the water, which causes a healing response, but the response of the organism to the application of heat or cold to the skin.

Philosophically, the science and art of hydrotherapy includes not only the application of water in its various forms, but also thermic application made by means of air, vapor, heated or cooled objects, electricity, and light. The use of medicants (herbs, minerals, or other active compounds) in conjunction with the application of water, has been a part of hydrotherapy since the time of Hippocrates. Hydrotherapy is actually better described as "thermotherapy"--the treatment of disease by the application of hot and cold. Water (the medium) is invaluable in treating disease because of its ability to carry heat or cold (the message) to enhance the body's ability to heal by affecting the nervous, circulatory, endocrine, and musculoskeletal systems. When water (in its various forms and temperatures) comes into contact with the skin, millions of nerve endings in the skin are stimulated. There also exists, a reflexive relationship between the skin and various organs, i.e. cold applied to the face contracts the cerebral blood vessels. Even though water and heat (or cold) are very ordinary, used properly they can do considerable good and if applied improperly they can do considerable harm.

C.   Principles of Hydrotherapy

When applying hydrotherapy treatments, the therapist must be knowledgeable in the basic physical concepts concerning thermal energy, the physical properties of water (or medicants), the organ systems of the body, which are influenced by hydrotherapy, and the physiological effects produced by the various therapeutic procedures. The human body attempts to maintain a uniform or "normal" stability known as "homeostasis." Environmental influences can affect physiological processes within the human body. In hydrotherapy, the environment of the body is changed by the application of water at different temperatures and with different methods.

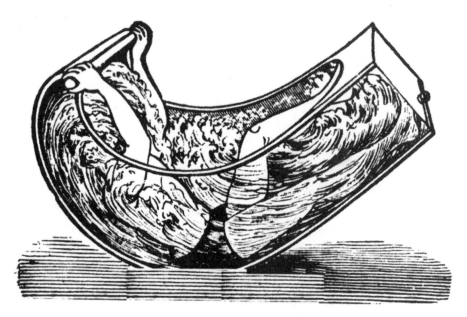

Primitive Manually Operated Whirlpool - Circa 1920

CHAPTER II SUMMARY - THEORY OF HYDROTHERAPY:

Definition: Hydrotherapy is defined as the application of water in its three forms (*solid, liquid, or vapor*) to the body, either externally or internally, in the treatment of disease or trauma.

It is understood that the practice of hydrotherapy may also include the use of herbal and chemical preparations applied in conjunction with applications of water -- such as with the use of plasters, poultices, masks, wraps, and baths.

Philosophy: The goal of hydrotherapy is to normalize the quantity of blood circulating through a given area, during a given period of time, by manipulating factors effecting circulation.

Hydrotherapy philosophically includes not only the use of water in its various forms, but also thermic applications made by means of heated or cooled air, objects, and the use of electricity and light.

Principles: In hydrotherapy, the environment of the body is changed by the application of water at different temperatures and with different methods.

NOTES

The Bathhouse at Bath, England

III. THERMODYNAMICS

A. Heat

Heat is the kinetic energy of the molecules within a substance and is defined in physics as the transfer of energy from one substance to another. Kinetic energy depends on the movement of molecules (atoms, nuclei, and electrons) in relationship to the temperature of the substance. For example, as the energy level of a substance increases, the movement of its molecules increases. When the physical state of a substance, such as water, is transformed, energy is released or stored as heat.

Heat is also defined as the amount of thermal energy of an object. The temperature of a particular object depends upon the number of particles within that object.

Heat is produced because of the difference in temperature between the two physical states. Heat is energy in "transit." Heat always flows from the substance at a higher temperature to the substance at a lower temperature. Usually this transfer raises the temperature of the substance receiving the heat, and lowers the temperature of the substance releasing the heat.

B. Temperature

Temperature is defined as the sensation of warmth or coldness of a substance on contact. Although we perceive the sensation of warmth or coldness, we cannot accurately measure this sensation without the use of scales. As the temperature of a substance varies, so does its physical properties. The substance expands or contracts and can change forms as well as exert varying pressures. This variation in properties usually serves as a basis for an accurate numerical temperature scale. Temperature is also dependant on the kinetic energy of the molecular motion.

Temperature is also defined as a measure of the average thermal energy of the particles within an object. It does not depend upon the number (or the size) of particles in that object.

C. Temperature Scales

Temperature is not heat but the *measurement* of the amount or level of heat. Thermometers measure the intensity of heat. There are five different temperature scales in use today--the Celsius known as Centigrade scale, the Fahrenheit scale, the Kelvin scale, the Rankine scale, and the International Thermodynamic Temperature scale. The Centigrade scale is widely used throughout the world, particularly in the scientific community. The Fahrenheit scale, developed by German physicist Daniel Fahrenheit, and used primarily in English-speaking countries, is based on the mercury thermometer.

The Centigrade and Fahrenheit scales are divided into 100 or 180 steps respectively, which define the freezing and the boiling point of water. The Centigrade scale simply divides the temperature range from freezing to boiling into 100 degrees. The Fahrenheit scale divides this same temperature range into 180 degrees. Freezing occurs at 0 degrees centigrade and 32 degrees Fahrenheit; boiling occurs at 100 degrees Centigrade or 212 degrees Fahrenheit. The centigrade degree is larger, being 9/5 the size of the Fahrenheit degree, or the Fahrenheit degree is 5/9 the size of the centigrade degree. To change Centigrade to Fahrenheit, one must first multiply by 9/5. This gives the number of Fahrenheit degrees above the freezing point. Since 32 is the freezing point on the Fahrenheit scale, it must then be added to the result to obtain the correct Fahrenheit reading. To change Fahrenheit to Centigrade, subtract 32 and multiply the remainder by 5/9 or:

Fahrenheit to Centigrade degrees = 5/9 or .555 x (Fahrenheit degrees - 32)
Centigrade to Fahrenheit degrees = 9/5 or 1.8 x Centigrade degrees (+ 32)

The following conversion table compares the two systems of temperature measurement. The practicing hydrotherapist should give careful attention to detail with regard to this measurement and documentation of temperature of both the treatment application and the patient.

Temperature Conversion Table

Celsius	Fahrenheit	
100°	212°	Boiling Point of Water
42	107.6	
41.5	106.7	Left Ventricle of Heart
41	105.8	Right Ventricle of Heart
40.5	104.9	
40	104.0	Normal Brain Temperature
39.5	103.1	
39	102.2	Normal Blood Temperature
38.5	101.3	
38	100.4	
37.5	99.6	Normal Rectal Temperature
37	98.6	Normal Oral Temperature
36.5	97.7	Normal Axillary Temperature
36	96.8	
35.5	95.9	
35	95.0	
34.5	94.0	Average Skin Temperature
0	32.0	Freezing Point of Water

Any references to temperature in this text will be Fahrenheit readings unless otherwise specified.

D. Heat Units

Heat is measured in terms of the ***calorie***. One calorie is defined as the amount of heat necessary to raise the temperature of one gram of pure water, at a pressure of one atmosphere, one degree on the centigrade scale. This unit is sometimes called the "small" or gram calorie (to distinguish it from the "large" calorie, or kilocalorie, which is often spoken of in nutrition and which is equal to 1,000 small or gram calories).

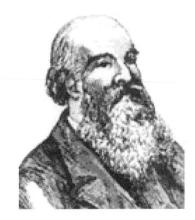

James Prescott Joule

Heat is also measured in quantities called joules in the metric system. The joule unit is named for the English physicist James P. Joule (1818-1889). He demonstrated that 4.19 joules of work are required to raise the temperature of 1 gram of water 1 degree centigrade.

E. Latent Heat

Substances exist in solid, liquid, or gaseous states. The process of changing from solid to gas is referred to as sublimation, from solid to liquid as melting, and from liquid to gas as vaporization. These changes occur at definite temperatures and pressures. If the pressure is constant, these processes occur at constant temperature. The amount of heat required to produce a change in state is called latent heat.

F. Specific Heat

Specific heat (heat capacity) is the measure of the amount of heat required to raise the temperature of a substance one degree. If the heating process occurs while the substance is maintained at a constant volume or is subjected to a constant pressure, the measure is referred to as a specific heat at constant volume or at constant pressure. (This will be discussed further in the section Properties of Water.)

G. Transfer of Heat

Heat is transferred from a higher temperature to a lower one. This transfer occurs through radiation, conduction, convection, evaporation, and conversion. In a warm-blooded creature, homeostasis attempts to balance the heat produced with the heat lost.

Radiation is the process where an object gives off or takes on thermal energy. Radiation does not require matter to accomplish the transfer of heat. A heat lamp uses radiation. Thermal radiation describes the electromagnetic radiation emitted from the surface of a body (which occurs primarily in the infrared band). If the external environment is cooler, heat will radiate from the skin into the cooler air. A nude person in a room at normal room temperature loses about 60% of his total heat loss by radiation, in the form of infrared heat rays. This loss increases as the temperature of the surroundings decreases.

Conduction is a method of heat transfer, which occurs when objects touch. It is a slow process. Only minute quantities of heat are lost from the body by direct conduction from the surface of the body to objects such as a chair or bed. However, loss of heat to air by conduction comprises a large portion of a body's heat loss. Skin and subcutaneous fat slow down the rate of heat conduction from the body's surface. Heat is conducted from the deep tissues of the body into the vascular system. From the body's core, it is carried from the deep circulatory system into the peripheral circulatory system, bringing warm blood to the surface. Conductive heat exchange increases as the difference between the skin and air temperature increases and as the amount of surface area involved increases. Paraffin baths, hot packs, and cold packs use the process of conduction to transfer heat.

Convection is a method of heat transfer in which the heated molecules move from one place to another. This is a more rapid transfer than conduction and occurs in liquids and gases. Within the human body, heat is first conducted into the air. The movement of the heated air is known as convection. A nude person seated in a comfortable room loses about 12 % of his heat by convection. The major means of transferring heat from the core of the body to the surface is by convection. Fluidotherapy uses convection--by blowing warm air over the patient's limbs. Another common example is the convection oven, in which super heated air passes over food.

Conversion is a form of heat transfer related to radiation and occurs when heat is generated in a substance or tissue as energy changes forms. Ultrasound, infrared lamps, and diathermy devices heat tissue via this process. For example, the high frequency sound waves of ultrasound, the low frequency light of infrared, and the electromagnetic waves of diathermy are "converted" to heat within the body's tissues.

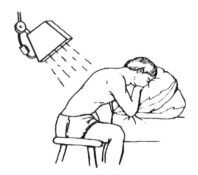

Radiation
(Infrared Lamp)

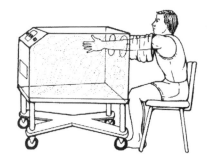

Convection
(Fluidotherapy)

CHAPTER III SUMMARY - THERMODYNAMICS:

Heat:	Heat is energy in transit, flowing from higher to lower energetic state.
Temperature:	Temperature is defined as the sensation of warmth or coldness of a substance on contact (not heat, but the measurement of heat).
Temperature Scales:	Centigrade and Fahrenheit scales are divided into 100 or 180 steps. respectively, which define the freezing and the boiling point of water (water freezes at 0 degrees Centigrade & 32 degrees Fahrenheit, water boils at 100 degrees Centigrade & 212 degrees Fahrenheit).
Heat Units:	Heat is measured in terms of the *calorie*. One calorie is defined as the amount of heat necessary to raise the temperature of one gram of pure water, at a pressure of one atmosphere, one degree on the centigrade scale.
Latent Heat:	The amount of heat required to produce a change in state is called latent heat.
Specific Heat:	Specific heat is the measure of the amount of heat required to raise the temperature of a substance one degree.
Transfer of Heat:	Heat is transferred from a higher temperature to a lower one. This Transfer occurs through radiation, conduction, convection, evaporation, and conversion.
Radiation:	Radiation is the process where an object gives off or takes on thermal energy. A heat lamp uses radiation. Thermal radiation describes the electromagnetic radiation emitted from the surface of a body (which occurs primarily in the infrared band).
Conduction:	Conduction is the method of heat transfer which occurs when objects touch (*water is a better "conductor" than air*).
Convection:	Convection is a method of heat transfer in which the heated molecules move from one place to another. This is a rapid form of transfer and occurs in liquids and gases (*as in a "convection" oven*).
Conversion:	Conversion is a form of heat transfer related to radiation and occurs when heat is generated in a substance or tissue as energy changes forms (*as in the conversion of "ultrasound" or "light" waves to heat*).

NOTES

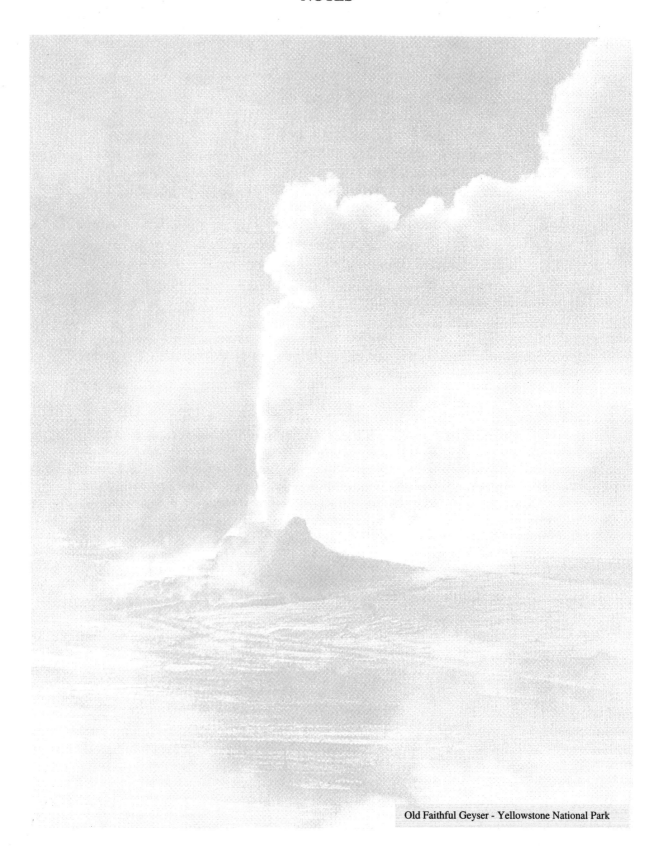

Old Faithful Geyser - Yellowstone National Park

IV. PROPERTIES OF WATER

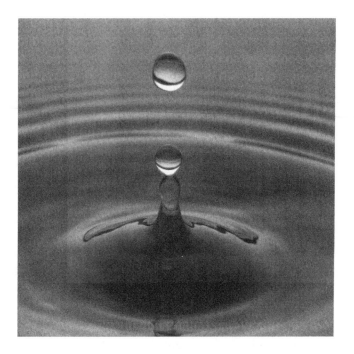

Water is abundant, affordable, available, easily applied, and provides buoyancy. The temperature and pressure of water are easily controlled. Water has several other properties, which make it an effective medium for hydrotherapy treatments.

Water exists in the **three states** of **solid** (ice), **liquid** (water) and **vapor** (steam) within a relatively narrow temperature range. It is an excellent **conductor**, which allows it to transfer heat effectively and quickly. Water is considered to be the **universal solvent**, capable of holding many substances in solution and can easily pass through tissues. Blood and most drinkable fluids are solutions containing primarily water.

Water has a high specific heat, meaning it can give up and absorb large quantities of heat. Water absorbs more heat for a given weight than any other substance and as such is the standard of "specific heat", meaning the specific heats of other substances are measured against water's specific heat. A large amount of heat is required to raise the temperature of water, and when it cools, water releases a large amount of heat.

When water is boiled in an open container at a pressure of one atmosphere, the temperature does not rise above 212 degrees F, no matter how much heat is applied. The heat that is absorbed without changing the temperature is latent heat. It is not lost, but is expended in changing the water to steam and stored in steam as energy. This latent energy is released when the steam is condensed to form water again. If a mixture of water and ice is heated, the water's temperature will not change until all the ice is melted. The latent heat absorbed is used up in overcoming the forces holding the particles of ice together and is stored as energy in the water. One gram of water at 80 degrees C would require a heat loss of approximately 160 calories before it would turn into ice. 80 calories of heat would be used to get the water to 0 degrees C (freezing point), and an additional 80 calories of *latent heat* would have to be used for it to become ice. This is significant to hydrotherapy because if freezing water gives off large quantities of latent heat then melting ice absorbs large quantities of latent heat. This makes ice a powerful tool for treatment.

Conversely, heat of vaporization is the energy necessary to evaporate a given liquid. It takes 540 calories per gram of water to change it from a liquid to a vapor. This process means that although it takes one calories to heat a gram of water from 99 to 100 degrees C, it takes 540 calories to turn that gram of 100 degree C water into steam. This explains why a serious burn may occur if water vapor condenses as steam on the skin. When the steam condenses, it gives off 540 times as much heat as would be given off when it cools from 100 to 99 degrees C. This concept is important for use of the Russian bath in hydrotherapy treatments. Much more heat is given off as the steam condenses, versus the temperature of the steam. Therefore, let's examine what happens when one gram of ice is heated to steam and then returned to form ice again. When heated, ice stores 80 calories of heat to become water; it then stores 540 calories of heat when changing to steam; it then loses the 540 calories on condensation; and finally, it loses the 80 calories on freezing. Because water has such a high specific heat, it is a powerful medium as a liquid. However, when it freezes and melts, it is 80 times more powerful. When the body is rubbed with ice, there is marked cooling of the body because actual heat transfers from the body to the ice, being stored in the melted water as latent heat. When the water vaporizes and condenses, it is 540 times more powerful.

Water is **fluid** and is easily applied. By using baths and compresses, water can be delivered and applied to the contour of all body parts. Water also has the ability to **conduct** heat to and away from the body rapidly. It carries heat to and from the body over 25 times faster than air. Good conductors, such as water, also feel hotter or colder than other materials (paper or plastic) that are not good conductors.

Water's density is very similar to that of the human body, which accounts for the buoyant effect when a body is immersed into a water tank and making it valuable in many forms of physical therapy. Water weighs eight pounds per gallon, and one cubic foot of water contains eight gallons. Therefore, the weight of one cubic foot of water is 64 pounds. The **hydrostatic pressure** or force of water is exerted evenly on the entire body surface, providing support, as well as resistance, when the body is immersed. Because of the physical properties of water, a larger volume of water will exert greater force or pressure against a body or body part. **Buoyancy** is the upward force generated by a liquid enabling submerged objects to have decreased apparent weight compared to their weight on land. Buoyancy acts opposite the force of gravity, resulting in an off-loading which helps in neuromuscular re-education. Because the weight of the limb being moved is much less, the affected muscles are now able to move the weight of the limb without undue stress. The decreased weight bearing can be measured in humans in relation to the level of their body that has been submerged. Approximately 90% of body weight is off-loaded when a human is submerged to the level of their neck.

Water is a polar molecule, allowing it to be a polar solvent. Water is the solvent found in biological systems. Its chemical structure (hydrogen bond) contributes to the stability of many biological structures (proteins & genetic components) within the human body. Water is generally considered to be a non-electrolyte (pH 7). However, 1 molecule in 10 million ionizes to produce a hydrogen (+) ion and a hydroxide (OH^-) ion component.

CHAPTER IV SUMMARY - PROPERTIES OF WATER:

Water: Abundant, affordable, available, easily applied & provides "buoyancy."

Exists in 3 states within a narrow (0 –100 C) temperature range
(*solid, liquid & vapor*).

Universal solvent (holds many varied solutes in solution).

Excellent conductor and has a high specific heat (easily takes on & gives up large amounts of energy).

Hydrostatic Pressure: The force exerted by water in all directions (evenly) against a body
The pressure exerted by a fluid is proportional to the density of that fluid and it's depth.

Buoyancy: Buoyancy is the upward force generated by a liquid enabling submerged objects to have decreased apparent weight compared to their weight on land.

Specific heat: Water has a high specific heat, meaning it can give up and absorb large quantities of heat. Water absorbs more heat for a given weight than any other substance, and as such is the standard of specific heat.

Hydrogen Bond: Type of bond that forms between the hydrogen (+) in one water molecule and the oxygen (-) of other water molecules.

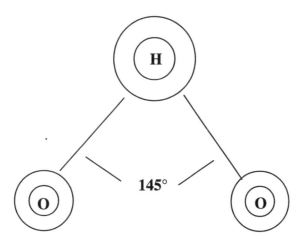

Polar Water Molecule

26

NOTES

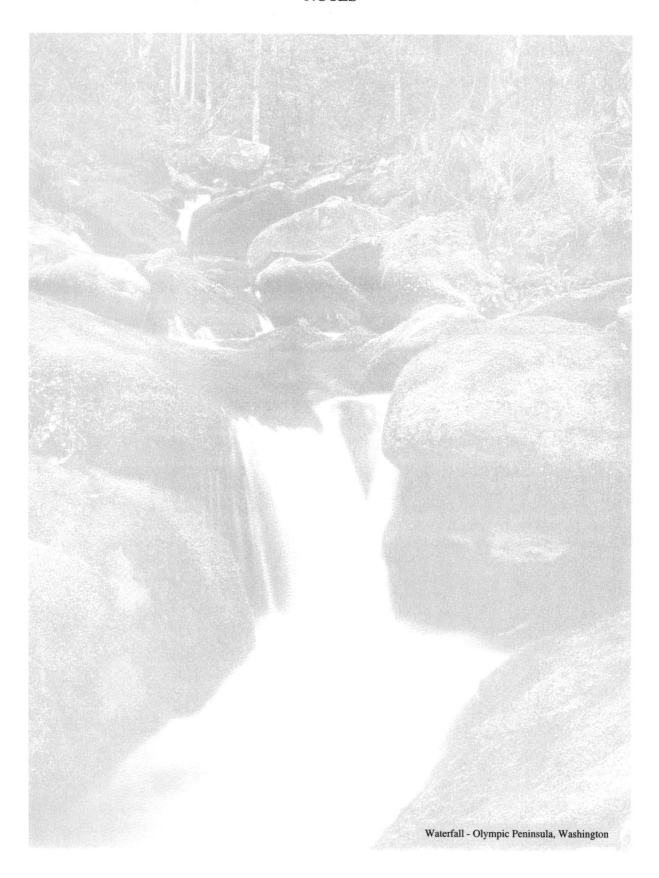

Waterfall - Olympic Peninsula, Washington

V. HUMAN ANATOMY AND PHYSIOLOGY

Anatomy is the branch of science that studies the form and structure of body parts. Physiology is the study of the function of these parts and systems. Each system of the body is affected by hydrotherapy. An understanding of the structure and function of the systems is necessary in order to understand the functional changes, which may occur from the use of hydrotherapy. Those body systems which are most influenced by hydrotherapy are the circulatory, nervous, endocrine, integumentary, muscular, and digestive. A brief review of those systems follows.

A. The Circulatory System

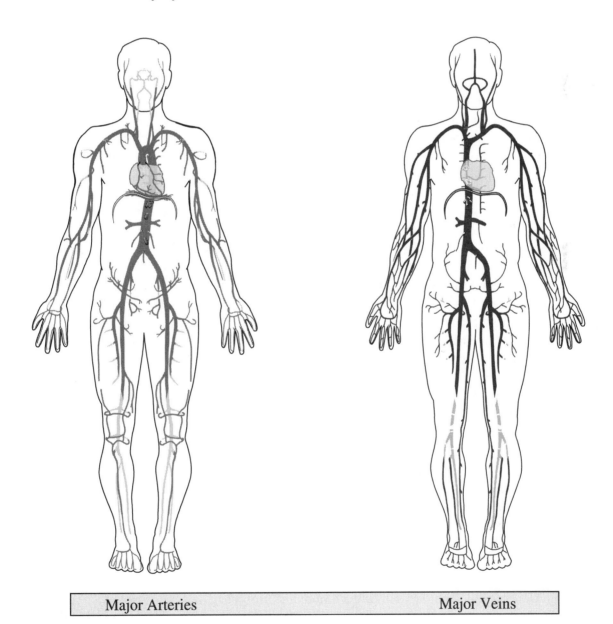

| Major Arteries | Major Veins |

The circulatory system, also referred to as cardiovascular system, includes the heart and a closed system of blood vessels consisting of arteries, arterioles, capillaries, venules, veins, and of the blood. The heart acts as a muscular pump which forces blood through the blood vessels. The blood serves as a fluid for transporting gases, nutrients, hormones, enzymes, and wastes. The circulatory system functions as a transport for blood between the body cells and various organs, which are connected with the external environment. The circulatory system is vital to our survival, supplying necessary oxygen and nutrients to all tissue cells, as well as removing waste substances, which have formed in the cells and tissues.

The heart is a four chambered muscular pump located within the thoracic cavity. It is generally about the size of a closed fist and is found just behind the body of the sternum, bounded on each side by the lungs, posteriorly by the spine and its lower edge (apex) rests on the diaphragm. The heart contains two atria and two ventricles, which function as two distinct pumps. The right side of the heart receives blood low in oxygen. Contractions of the right atria and ventricle push the blood to the lungs via the pulmonary arteries, where carbon dioxide molecules and wastes are released from the blood and oxygen is absorbed. The freshly oxygenated blood then returns to the left side of the heart via the pulmonary veins. This route of blood flow is known as pulmonary circulation. The blood then passes through the left side of the heart, exiting through the aorta for transport throughout the body. Blood is supplied to the muscle tissue of the heart by the first two branches of the aorta known as the right and left coronary arteries.

Arteries are strong, elastic blood vessels, well adapted to carry blood away from the heart under high pressure. All arteries, except the pulmonary arteries, carry oxygen-rich (oxygenated) blood. The aorta is the largest artery in the body; it extends up from the left ventricle, arches over the heart to the left and descends just in front of the vertebral column. The aorta then divides into somewhat smaller arteries, which subdivide into gradually thinner tubes and end in fine branches called arterioles. These small arteries carry blood from the artery to the capillaries, which are only one cell thick, making them the only vessels capable of exchanging gases and nutrients between the blood and body cells. Although the capillaries are microscopic (only 1/25 " long), if joined together, they would measure 62,000 miles in length. Once cubic inch of muscle has 1.5 million capillaries. No cell in the body is far removed from a capillary. It is important to know that a partial cuff of smooth muscle on the arteriole, the *precapillary sphincter*, controls blood flow to the capillaries by expanding and contracting. It is of great importance for maintaining normal blood pressure and circulation, and is noticeably influenced by hydrotherapy. The capillaries connect the smallest arterioles to the smallest venules, which then merge to form larger veins. Veins are composed primarily of connective tissue with some muscular and elastic tissue. They function to carry blood toward the heart. All veins, except the pulmonary veins coming from the lungs, carry oxygen-poor (deoxygenated) blood. An important anatomical feature of veins is their valves, which prevent the back-flow of blood and aid in returning blood back to the heart. As the veins reach the heart, they become very large and are known as the superior and inferior vena cavae. (Veins hold about two times the amount of blood as arteries). The vena cavae, which are the largest of veins, empty the oxygen-poor blood into the right atrium, completing the part of blood flow known as the systemic circulation.

Blood is the semi-liquid fluid, which courses through the circulatory system. It contains billions of formed (solid) elements known as blood cells in a liquid medium known as plasma. The total blood volume varies greatly with age, sex, and body type. Blood volume per kilogram varies inversely with the amount of excess body fat. A healthy male might average 71 ml. of blood per kilogram of body weight. This means a 70 kilogram or 150 lb. male would average 5,000 ml. or 5 quarts of blood. Of the total blood volume, 55% is plasma; the remaining 45% is formed elements. Plasma consists mainly (91%) of water with a variety of dissolved materials. Cellular products such as hormones, enzymes, and urea are transported in the plasma, as are electrolytes, proteins, fats, sugars, and gases (oxygen, nitrogen and carbon dioxide).

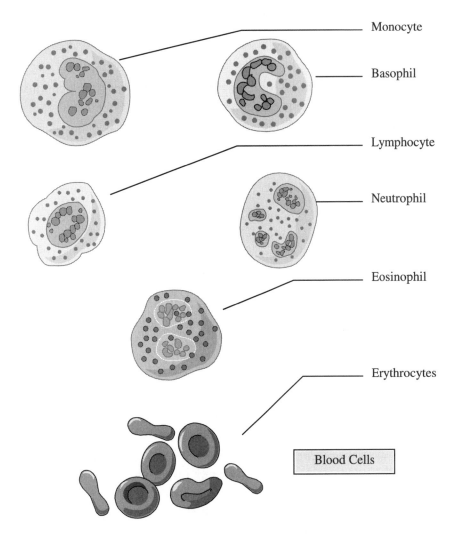

Monocyte

Basophil

Lymphocyte

Neutrophil

Eosinophil

Erythrocytes

Blood Cells

The formed element portion of the blood includes erythrocytes (red blood cells), leukocytes (white blood cells), and thrombocytes (platelets). Of the formed elements, erythrocytes are by far the most numerous. They are small (5 million in a cubic millimeter of blood) bi-concave circular discs, which contain a substance called hemoglobin, capable of combining with large quantities of oxygen and carbon dioxide. Erythrocytes (RBCs) are formed in red bone marrow and live about 120 days in circulation. They are then destroyed by the liver and spleen, and their parts recycled. Hormones control the number of circulating RBCs. (Anemia is the condition in which too little oxygen is carried to tissue cells by the RBCs.)

Leukocytes or white blood cells are additional formed elements present in the blood. They are fewer in number (but larger in size) than the RBCs. They are also formed by the red bone marrow but mature in different sites throughout the body, such as the liver, spleen, and thymus. As a group, leukocytes (WBCs) guard against invasion of foreign organisms and chemicals, and remove debris resulting from the death or injury of other cells. WBCs are also found outside the boundaries of the circulatory system. There are five major types of leukocytes (lymphocytes, monocytes, neutrophils, eosinophils, and basophils). Each plays a particular role in the defense of our bodies. All WBCs are motile (they can move).

Neutrophils and monocytes actually eat and digest microbes (a process known as phagocytosis). Eosinophils are weak phagocytes but are limited in their motility. They usually function to detoxify proteins and other harmful products, which result from allergic reactions and infections by parasites. Most types of WBCs easily move out of the capillaries into tissue by squeezing through the intercellular spaces of the capillary walls by a process known as *diapedesis*.

Basophils are not phagocytes, but release chemicals into the blood stream and tissue that will increase the permeability of the capillary walls. Basophils are related to mast cells, which reside in connective tissue and are responsible for the release of the inflammatory chemical, histamine. Monocytes are known also as tissue macrophages, and are large phagocytic cells associated with the inflammatory response.

Lymphocytes are primarily found in lymphatic structures such as the lymph nodes, liver, spleen, and tonsils. Lymphocytes are primarily responsible for the production of antibodies. *Chemotaxis* is the name given to the attraction of WBCs to an inflamed area. It is believed that a large group of chemicals including bacterial toxins, kinins, histamines, clotting factors, and "complement complex" products actually draw white blood cells to the area of inflammation. When inflammation is present, we can be assured that WBCs are at work. The cardinal characteristics of inflammation include: **pain**, **heat**, **redness,** and **swelling**. Redness and heat are explained by the increased blood flow. Swelling results from increased blood vessel permeability. The effects of kinins, prostaglandins, and other neurotransmitters on nerve endings produce pain.

Numerous studies have demonstrated that both diapedesis and chemotaxis increase with increases in tissue temperature.

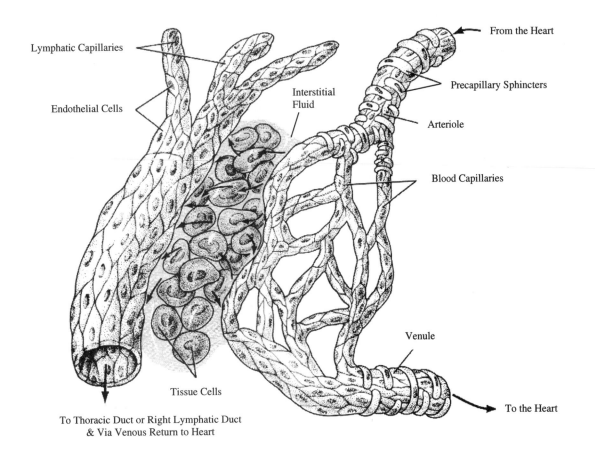

Lymphatic Capillaries

Endothelial Cells

Interstitial Fluid

From the Heart

Precapillary Sphincters

Arteriole

Blood Capillaries

Venule

Tissue Cells

To the Heart

To Thoracic Duct or Right Lymphatic Duct
& Via Venous Return to Heart

The lymphatic system is closely related to the circulatory system. Fluid (plasma), which leaks from the blood capillaries, accumulates between tissue cells, and is known as interstitial fluid. Some of this fluid leaves the interstitial spaces through a series of lymphatic capillaries to become lymph. The lymphatic system contains microscopic capillaries, which are very permeable, and a series of vein-like vessels that transport the lymph back to join the blood near the heart. Included in this system are a series of pea-sized filters known as lymph nodes. These nodes function to remove foreign substances from the lymph by phagocytosis, thereby preventing entry into the blood stream. Compared to normal circulatory blood flow, the flow of lymph is quite slow. Approximately two to four quarts of lymph are transported every 24 hours. This slow rate occurs because the lymphatic system (unlike the systemic circulation), has no pump. This system depends upon the "lymphatic pump" or contraction of skeletal muscle and the force of respiration to move lymphatic fluid back "uphill" to join the blood. Lymphatic flow is assisted by the intrinsic pumping (via myotatic reflex) of the visceral muscle within lymphatic vessel walls and by increased interstitial fluid pressure. The lymphatic vessels, nodes, and associated organs, (such as the liver, spleen, thymus and tonsils) thus serve to protect us by removing and destroying invaders and foreign particles before they can do harm. Specialized lymphatic capillaries called *lacteals* carry dietary fats from the digestion system to the blood stream.

B. The Nervous System

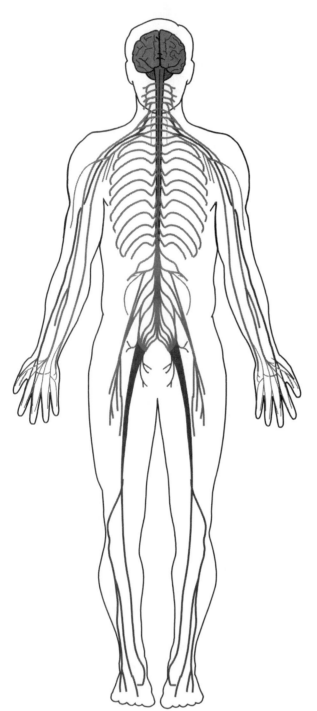

The nervous system consists of the brain, spinal cord and associated nerves. The brain and spinal cord comprise the Central Nervous System (CNS), which is completely encased within bony structures. The Peripheral Nervous System (PNS) is composed of nerves, which connect outlying parts of the body with the CNS. All of the PNS lies outside the cranial and spinal cavities. It functions to control and coordinate all body activities with rapid and precise actions. Some nerve cells are specialized to detect changes that occur inside and outside of the body. Other nerve cells receive these impulses, interpret them, and act on the information they receive. Still other nerve cells carry impulses from the brain or spinal cord to muscles or glands and stimulate these parts to contract or to secrete.

The brain is the largest and most complex part of the nervous system. It lies in the cranial cavity of the skull and is composed of billions of nerve cells and countless nerve fibers. The nerve cells communicate with one another and with nerve cells in other parts of the system. Each nerve cell, known as a *neuron*, consists of a main part called the *cell body*, one or more branch-like extensions known as *dendrites*, and one elongated projection known as an *axon*. The membrane of a neuron receives or initiates an impulse at the dendrite end and carries the message to the axon end to stimulate another neuron or a tissue cell. In this way, messages are received and are rapidly acted upon by the brain.

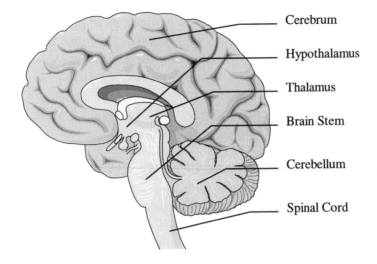

Cerebrum

Hypothalamus

Thalamus

Brain Stem

Cerebellum

Spinal Cord

The brain consists of the following four major divisions: cerebrum; cerebellum; diencephalon and brain stem. The cerebrum is the largest and uppermost part of the brain, consisting of two large lobes, which are mirror images of each other. The cerebrum is involved with conscious thought, willed movements, sensory perceptions, emotions, and memory. The cerebellum, second largest part of the human brain, is located below the cerebrum and lies in the posterior section of the cranial cavity. The cerebellum functions to coordinate skeletal muscle movement, equilibrium, and posture. The diencephalon is a small, but important part of the brain, located between the cerebrum above and the midbrain below, consisting of two major structures, the *hypothalamus* and the *thalamus*. ***The hypothalamus is the temperature-regulating center of the body.*** Specialized temperature-sensing neurons within the hypothalamus respond to temperature changes of the blood by becoming more active or less active. The diencephalon is involved with sensation and emotion at an unconscious level such as regulation of body temperature, water balance, sleep, appetite, and sexual arousal. It is known as our "regulatory center." The brain stem is a bundle of nerve tissue that extends downward from the base of the cerebrum to the level of the spinal cord. The brain stem consists of the midbrain, pons, and medulla oblongata; and is concerned with vital functions - respiration, heartbeat, vision, auditory impulses, and vasomotor control. The medulla oblongata is an extension of the spinal cord and is a two-way conduction pathway between the spinal cord and higher brain centers.

The spinal cord is a slender nerve column, which extends downward from the brain stem through the vertebral canal to the bottom of the first lumbar vertebra. The spinal cord contains thousands and thousands of nerve cells, which conduct impulses between the brain and all parts of the body. It is the primary reflex center of the body. The center core of the spinal cord consists mainly of dendrites and cell bodies of neurons, which receive information. Bundles of nerve fibers called spinal tracts surround this inner core. These spinal tracts provide a two-way conduction path to and from the brain. Ascending tracts conduct impulses up the cord to the brain, whereas descending tracts conduct impulses down the cord from the brain. Spinal tracts transmit impulses that produce sensations of *crude touch, pain, temperature,* and *pressure.* They also control many voluntary and involuntary movements.

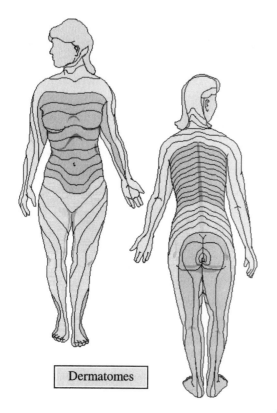

Dermatomes

Twelve pairs of cranial nerves arise from various locations on the under surface of the brain and lead to parts of the head, neck, and trunk. These cranial nerve fibers are associated with the sense of smell, vision, eye movements, hearing, taste, and general sense of movements of the face and jaw.

There are thirty-one pairs of nerves, which arise from the spinal cord. These spinal nerves exit from the spinal cord and branch to form the many outlying nerves of the trunk and limbs. They conduct impulses between the spinal cord and the parts of the body not supplied by cranial nerves. The skin segment supplied by a single spinal nerve is called a **dermatome**. Dermatomes provide a "map" of specific nerve activity. The nerves that carry nerve impulses from outer (peripheral) parts of the body into the brain or spinal cord are known as *sensory (afferent)* neurons.

Changes, which occur inside or outside of the body, such as temperature, stimulate these cells to send a message to the brain or spinal cord. Upon receiving this message, other nerve cells are acted upon to respond to such changes. Nerves that carry messages from the brain or spinal cord to other parts of the body are known as *motor (efferent)* neurons. When motor impulses reach muscles, for example, the muscle cells are either stimulated to contract or to relax. When these impulses reach glands, the gland is stimulated to release or reduce its secretions. Sensory and motor impulses travel through different nerve fibers within the same cranial or spinal nerve. The specialized senses, such as smell, taste, hearing, and sight, travel to the brain via the cranial nerves. Most other senses send impulses to the CNS via the sensory neurons of the spinal nerve segments. As mentioned above, this dermatomal distribution demonstrates the relationship between various organs, glands, tissues, and specific nerve pathways.

The peripheral nervous system includes pathways that carry impulses from the CNS to peripheral structures of the body and pathways by which sensory impulses from peripheral structures reach the CNS. Included in the PNS are the cranial and spinal nerves and their distal fibers. Functionally, the PNS is divided into: (1) the Sensory Nervous System whose (afferent) fibers carry impulses from sense receptors to the CNS, (2) the Somatic Nervous System whose (efferent) fibers carry impulses from the CNS to skeletal muscle, and (3) the Autonomic Nervous System whose (efferent) fibers carry impulses from the CNS to visceral (smooth) muscle, cardiac muscle, and glandular (secretory) tissue.

In response to both internal changes in the body and those of the external environment, the Autonomic Nervous System relays impulses to organs, glandular tissue, and visceral muscle to compensate and maintain homeostasis. The ANS is separated into two distinct divisions, the sympathetic (thoracolumbar) and the parasympathetic (craniosacral). As a general rule, these two divisions have opposing functions. Most of the organs, glands, and visceral muscle are innervated by both divisions of the ANS. Generally, the stimulation of one division increases the activity of an organ, while stimulation of the other decreases it. Through the regulatory activity of the hypothalamus, a balance exists between the activities of the Sympathetic and Parasympathetic divisions. When viewed in general terms, the Sympathetic division prepares the organs for emergency situations, such as required during aggressive or defensive behavior. This is commonly known as the "**Fight or Flight**" response. These reactions include increased heart rate, increased blood flow to skeletal muscle, dilation of bronchi, dilation of pupils of the eye, vasoconstriction in the skin and extremities, and cessation of digestive functions. In contrast, the Parasympathetic division maintains the various organs at activity levels commensurate with maintaining normal internal homeostasis of the body.

Specialized receptors are located throughout the body to transmit sensory data.

1. **Thermal receptors** for the perception of temperature change exist in many human body tissues. In most areas of the body, there exist 3 to 10 times as many receptors for cold as those for warmth. The specific number of receptors in different areas of the body varies; from 15 to 25 cold receptors per square centimeter in the lips, to 3 to 5 cold receptors per square centimeter in some broad areas of the torso. There exist correspondingly fewer numbers of warmth receptors. The numbers of these receptors appear to be consistent from person to person. Cold receptors appear to be much more rapid and efficient than warmth receptors. Subgroups of these thermal receptors include pain fibers that are stimulated by cold, cold fibers, warmth fibers, and pain fibers that are stimulated by heat. Theses receptors or fibers respond differently at different levels of temperature. This differentiation in response to stimuli allows a person to discriminate different gradations of thermal sensation. One can also understand why either extreme cold or extreme heat can elicit sensations of pain. Thermal receptors have been found to adapt rapidly to any given stimuli. Perception of cold or heat "fades" rapidly during the first 30 seconds of exposure and then more slowly for the next 30 minutes or longer. Thermal perception via these receptors is most notable therefore, to *changes in temperature.* Because the total number of cold or warmth receptors in any small area of the body is relatively few, it is difficult to judge slight temperature changes when that small area alone is stimulated. When a large area of the body is stimulated, thermal signals are combined to elicit a stronger sensation in a process known as *"summation."* The human body can therefore detect temperature changes as small as .01 degree C when temperature affects the entire body surface. Temperature changes 100 times this great might not be perceived if only one square centimeter of surface were exposed.

2.   **Baroreceptors** for measuring arterial blood pressure are located in the Aorta.

3.   Various **mechanoreceptors** are located in integumentary tissue for registering **pressure, crude touch, fine touch, vibration** (tactile sensations), and **proprioception** (position). The best-known proprioceptors are the *Muscle Spindle Cells* and the *Golgi Tendon Organs*.

4.   **Chemoreceptors** are located in the aorta for measuring carbon dioxide, and in the hypothalamus for measuring amounts of hormones, enzymes, proteins, blood glucose, amino acids, fats, etc.

5.   **Nociceptors** are located in various tissues to register pain. All pain receptors or nociceptors are known to exist as free nerve endings. They are widespread in superficial layers of the skin as well as in certain internal tissues, such as periosteum, arterial walls, joint surfaces, and portions of the cranial vault. Most other deep structures contain notably fewer pain receptors. Any widespread tissue damage can nonetheless elicit chronic, aching pain sensations arising from these tissues. Nociceptors exist in three forms and are stimulated by *mechanical, thermal,* or *chemical* stimuli. In contrast to other types of receptors, nociceptors adapt little (or not at all) to continued stimuli. In fact, excitation of pain fibers appears to become progressively greater with continued stimulation (facilitation). Pain sensations initiated by any of the above types of fibers tends to correspond directly to tissue destruction and intensity of pain perceived tends to correspond to the rate and amount of tissue damage occurring. It is postulated that *ischemia* (hypoxia) is the major contributing factor leading to cell dysfunction, cell death (necrosis), tissue damage, and therefore pain.

In response to information received from these varied receptors, the CNS integrates responses, which include endocrine gland stimulation as well as both Somatic and Autonomic Nervous System stimulation. Both reflex and conscious responses are transmitted from the CNS through either the Somatic or Autonomic nervous systems to appropriate target organs, glands, and muscle. In this manner, precise and rapid control over all body functions is coordinated.

Of special interest is the fact that thermal signals are transmitted in nearly parallel and adjacent pathways to pain signals. Thermal signals terminate in the brainstem, the thalamus or the sensory cortex of the cerebrum. It is well documented that competitive stimulation (tactile, thermal, chemical, or electrical) may depress the transmission or recognition of pain (noxious) signals. Melzack and Wall first described this phenomenon in 1965 as the "Gate-Control Hypothesis" or hyperstimulation analgesia. Later work by Parsons and Goetzl demonstrated that using a vapo-coolent (counterirritant) produced significant local pain reduction. Recent research by Bini, et al, has also demonstrated that stimulation of cold sensitive receptors depressed pain at the segmental level. Subsequent studies have documented that all nerve cell transmissions are altered by relatively slight changes in local tissue temperature.

C. The Endocrine System

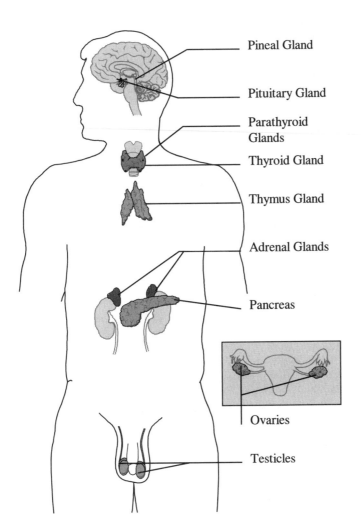

Pineal Gland

Pituitary Gland

Parathyroid Glands

Thyroid Gland

Thymus Gland

Adrenal Glands

Pancreas

Ovaries

Testicles

The endocrine system is composed of various glands, which include the pituitary, thyroid, parathyroid, adrenal, pineal, and thymus glands; as well as the pancreas, ovaries, placenta, and testes. The term "endocrine" is used to describe glands that secrete their substances internally. Also, because they have no duct system, endocrine glands are also known as "ductless glands." All of these glands secrete chemicals called hormones. Hormones travel to all parts of the body in the blood. Usually, a particular hormone only affects a particular tissue, called its "target tissue." The effect of the hormone is to regulate in some way the function of this target tissue and therefore play a vital role in the control of metabolism. As a group, the endocrine glands function to control the rates of certain chemical reactions, aid in the transport of substances through cell membranes, regulate stress responses, play vital roles in cell growth, and help regulate water and electrolyte balance. As the nervous system transmits nerve impulses at a relatively rapid rate providing generally brief effects, the endocrine system exerts slower but longer-lasting control.

Endocrine glands release hormones and exert their influence on their target tissues in this way: the endocrine gland secrets its hormone(s); the hormone is carried to the target cell by body fluid; the hormone combines with its receiver site on the membrane of the target cell; molecules are then activated within the target cell's membrane and scatter out into the contents of the cell bringing about the desired cellular changes. The concentration of each hormone in the body fluids remains relatively constant. When an imbalance in hormone concentration occurs, this information is fed back to some part of the system that acts to correct this imbalance. Some endocrine glands secrete their hormones in response to nerve impulses, and others react in response to hormones which have been released from the hypothalamus and/or anterior pituitary.

Although not intended to present the workings of the endocrine system in great detail, a brief discussion of a few endocrine structures and their hormones is warranted.

The **pituitary gland** is directly influenced by the hypothalamus and in turn produces at least eight hormones. From the posterior pituitary *ADH (Anti-diuretic hormone)* plays an important role in regulating the water concentration of the body fluids. Increased levels of ADH influence the kidneys to reduce the amount of water secreted (urine). Both *GH (Growth Hormone)* and *TSH (Thyroid Stimulating hormone)* are produced by the anterior pituitary and influence the ultimate rate at which the body metabolizes fuel. GH influences the body's cells to increase in size and thus use more of all types of fuels (carbohydrates, fats, and proteins). TSH stimulates the thyroid gland, which in turn stimulates the rate of cellular metabolism.

The **pineal gland** is a small structure located deep within the brain and is attached directly to the thalamus. *Melatonin* is secreted by the pineal gland in response to light conditions outside the body. Information regarding the amount of light is transmitted to the pineal via the optic nerve. When the amount of light decreases, the pineal secretes more melatonin. The pineal is considered to be the body's internal clock, establishing our internal or *circadian* rhythms in response to changes in available light such as day and night. Sleep/wake cycles, migration of birds, and the fertility cycles of many mammals are dependent upon their pineal gland.

The **thyroid** gland is located just below the larynx in front of the trachea. The thyroid produces two hormones that have a direct effect on cellular metabolic rate. These hormones known as *T4* and *T3* both increase the rate at which cells convert sugars and fats into energy. A number of disorders are associated with hyper or hypo secretion of the thyroid hormones. The effects of these disorders include abnormalities of body temperature.

The **adrenal** glands, which are attached to the top of each kidney, produce a number of hormones. *Epinephrine (adrenaline)* and *nor-epinephrine* both exert an influence on the body that is similar (but longer lasting) to the sympathetic nervous system (Fight or Flight) response. The physiological effects include increased heart rate, elevated blood pressure, increased respiratory rate, and decreased digestive activity. This intense state may also increase core body temperature. *Aldosterone* is also produced by the adrenal glands. The action of aldosterone involves the regulation of fluid and electrolyte balance. An increase in aldosterone levels causes the kidneys (and sweat glands) to reabsorb sodium. As a consequence of this conservation, blood levels of sodium and chloride rise while potassium is unaffected and continues to be lost with urine and sweat. By saving sodium and chloride, water is indirectly conserved, thus causing increased blood volume and blood pressure. *Cortisol* from the adrenal cortex suppresses the immune response, and inflammation, while increasing blood sugar levels. Please review in a physiology text, the functions of the adrenal glands as they relate to the effects of stress.

Prostaglandins (also known as tissue hormones) are chemical compounds formed in specialized cells of many tissues such as the heart, blood vessels, skin, and bronchi. These chemicals do not enter the blood stream, as do other hormones, but move by diffusion to influence nearby tissues. Prostaglandins are thought to aid in the control of such functions as respiration, vasodilation, inflammation, and cardiac rhythm.

D. The Integumentary System

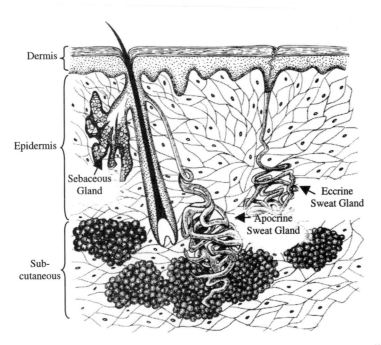

The integumentary complex is a sheet-like structure composed of the skin and its appendages. It comprises nearly 20 square feet of surface area and it varies in thickness from 1/50th to 1/8th of an inch. It is in fact the largest organ of the body. The crucial functions of the integument include protection, sensation, chemical production, and heat regulation. The integument is composed of two distinct tissue layers, the outer, thinner epidermis and the deeper, thicker dermis. Under the dermis is the subcutaneous tissue area containing both fibrous connective tissue (fascia) and adipose (fat).

The epidermis is less than 1/200th of an inch thick in most areas (the palms of the hands and soles of the feet are thicker). This layer of skin is composed of dead cells, which have been converted to the waterproof and chemical resistant protein substance, keratin, and millions of closely packed living cells. New keratinocytes are formed in a basal layer and migrate outward to die (keratinized) and eventually flake off (desquamate). The entire epidermis is replaced every two weeks.

Deep in the epidermis, interspersed between the keratinocytes, are specialized cells known as melanocytes. These cells produce the pigment (melanin) which gives skin its brown tone. The more melanin, the more brown the skin tone will be. UV light rays stimulate the production of melanin. While the keratinocytes provide physical protection from trauma and water loss, the melanocytes confer some protection to the underlying dermis from UV light (the epidermis contains no blood vessels).

The deeper and thicker dermis is a more complicated structure. It is composed primarily of fibrous connective tissue - tough collagen fibers, elastin fibers, and a gel-like ground substance. The dermis contains an abundant supply of blood vessels (capillaries) and nerve endings. Also contained in the dermis are sweat glands, sebaceous glands, hair follicles, and small muscles called the arrector pili. In fact, on the average, each square inch of skin contains over 500 sweat glands, 1,000 nerve endings, yards of capillaries, over 100 sebaceous glands, and hundreds of sensors (for pressure, heat, cold and pain).

The numerous capillaries of the skin are controlled by motor neurons originating in the central nervous system, thus regulating the amount of blood available to the dermis. Contraction of the arrector pili muscle causes goose bumps and is under the control of the central nervous system.

Sebaceous glands produce an oily substance "sebum" which is secreted through small ducts into the hair follicle keeping the hair and skin soft, flexible, and relatively water proof. Oil based substances enter the body more easily through the skin than do water based solutions which are virtually excluded. Sebaceous glands are absent from the palms of the hands, soles of the feet, and the lips.

Hair follicles have a rich supply of blood at their base, allowing for rapid cell proliferation. As cells mature and grow, they move toward the skin surface. The cells that move upward and away from their nutrient source become keratinized and die, forming the hair shaft, which extends above the skin surface. Nails have a similar origin as hair, but contain a denser version of keratin.

Sweat glands are found in nearly all regions of the skin in humans. They are more numerous in the skin of the palms and soles. Each gland consists of a very small tube, which originates as an oval or round-coiled structure deep in the dermis. The coiled portion is lined with specialized sweat secreting cells. The outer opening of the sweat gland is known as a pore. The sweat or "sudoriferous" glands are classified as either eccrine or apocrine.

Eccrine glands are most numerous and are found in the skin of almost all body areas. They function throughout life to produce a thick fluid consisting mainly of water with small quantities of sodium, chloride, potassium, urea, and uric acid. In subjects where liver and kidney function is diminished, sweat may become concentrated with compounds that the body is unable to excrete through normal processes. Decreased liver function increases blood concentration and the diffusion of elements and compounds from capillaries of skin into sweat glands. The secretion of sweat is therefore, to a limited degree, an excretory function.

Appocrine sweat glands are most numerous in the groin and axillary regions where they are usually connected to hair follicles. These glands secrete a thicker protein-rich fluid, which provides nourishment for bacteria and leads to the production of a characteristic odor. The apocrine glands are stimulated to secrete during times of emotional stress such as feelings of fear or pain. The development of these glands is stimulated by sex hormones and becomes functional as one reaches puberty.

There are several types of sensory receptors located in the skin, each being sensitive to one modality of sensation. Specialized receptors carry information regarding crude touch, fine touch, pressure, vibration, heat, cold, and pain. Those receptors for sensations such as pressure, touch, and vibration are classified as mechanoreceptors and those for pain are nociceptors. Unmyelinated neurons from pain and temperature receptors travel adjacent pathways in route to the brain.

The conversion of Vitamin D into its active form (D3), occurs in the skin with exposure to ultraviolet light. Research suggests that 20 minutes exposure several times a week is sufficient to provide adequate amounts of Vitamin D.

The subcutaneous layer lies below the dermis and is formed by loose connective and adipose tissue. Because the collagen and elastic tissues in this layer are continuous with those of the dermis, there exists no well-defined boundary between these two layers. The adipose tissue of the subcutaneous layer serves as insulation, thus excluding heat from the outside and conserving interior heat. It also allows skin considerable freedom of movement. Superficial fascia (subcutaneous tissue) is most distinct over the abdomen and is thinnest on the dorsal surfaces of the hands and feet. Fibrous connective tissue (yellow) of the hypodermis is primarily composed of elastin fibers, differing from the deep fascia, which is composed primarily of collagen fibers (white fibrous connective tissue). Fascial tissue is not only composed of protein-based fibers, but also a water-based substance called matrix. At higher temperatures, the matrix exhibits more solvent or fluid-like properties allowing a greater degree of elasticity. At lower temperatures, the matrix becomes more solid or gel-like, thus restricting both permeability and mobility.

E. The Muscular System

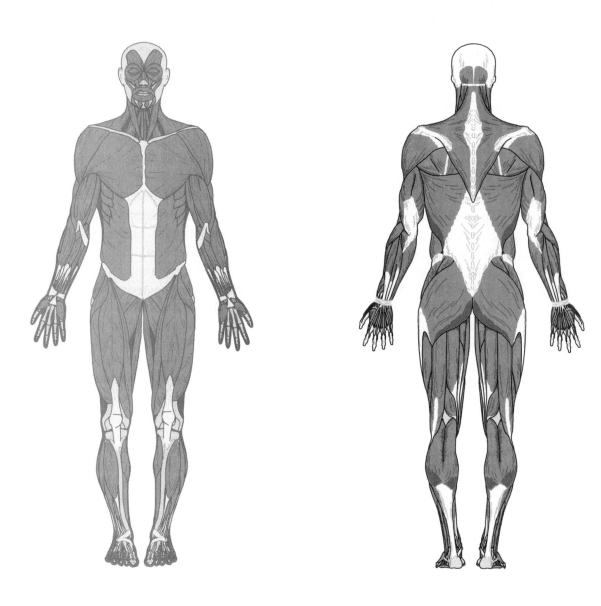

Anterior Muscles	Posterior Muscles

The muscular system consists of individual muscles, which are responsible for body movements, maintenance of posture, and generating heat. When muscle cells are stimulated, they contract and pull at their attachments, producing movement. Muscles account for nearly half of the body weight.

There are three types of muscle in the body: skeletal; visceral (smooth), and cardiac. Skeletal muscle is striated (striped) and is under voluntary control. It is attached to bones and functions to move these bones or to hold them in position. Visceral muscle is smooth (it does not have striations) and is found in the walls of internal organs providing the means for the organs to function. It is involuntary since it cannot be controlled by conscious thought. Cardiac muscle is striated, involuntary, and found in only one place in the body, the walls of the heart.

Skeletal muscle is attached to bones. Most skeletal muscles originate on one bone, cross a moveable joint, and attach on another bone. Movement is produced when the muscle contracts and pulls the movable bone to the more stationary bone. These contractions allow for movement of individual body parts or motion of the entire skeletal system, as in walking. The continued partial contraction of many skeletal muscles enables us to maintain posture as we sit or stand. Skeletal muscle is composed mainly of striated muscle cells and connective tissue, with smaller amounts of nerve and vascular tissue. Skeletal muscle cells are cylindrical in shape and contain many nuclei. Each muscle cell, known as a muscle fiber, is made up of protein fibers. The striations, or stripes, visible in skeletal muscle, are a result of the arrangement of its protein fibers. These threadlike protein structures, called myofilaments, are composed of a thick form of protein called myosin, and a thin form of protein known as actin. Myofilaments lie parallel to each other and continue through the length of the muscle fiber. Muscle fibers are grouped into bundles and are held together by a layer of connective tissue. These bundles, called fascicles, in turn, are grouped and held together by another layer of connective tissue eventually constructing a whole muscle.

Skeletal muscle fibers specialize in the function of contracting. To do so, a motor neuron from the central nervous system must transmit an impulse to the muscle. The area where this nerve ending nearly touches the muscle fiber is known as a neuromuscular junction. As the motor neuron comes in contact with the muscle fiber, a chemical called acetylcholine is released, stimulating the muscle fiber to contract. Energy and calcium are also required for a muscular contraction to occur. The energy supplied for muscular contraction comes from ATP molecules, which are produced within the cell. To produce ATP the cell needs fuel (primarily glucose) and oxygen. Both of these substances must be transported to the muscle by the blood. About 25% to 40 % of the fuel produced in a muscle cell is available to do work, the remainder becomes *heat*. As the muscle becomes more active, more heat is produced. Contraction occurs as the actin and myosin myofilaments slide towards each other pulling each contractile unit of the muscle, known as a sarcomere, closer together. Each single motor neuron, together with the muscle cells it interacts with is known as a motor unit. Depending on the need, different numbers of motor units may be activated for various loads. A muscle fiber will not contract until its stimulus reaches a certain level of intensity. The least amount of stimulation required for a muscle fiber to contract is known as its threshold stimulus. When a muscle fiber is adequately stimulated to contract, it will always contract completely.

Skeletal muscles are not only stimulated by nerve impulses. Although nerve impulses are the "natural" inducement for skeletal muscles to contract or relax, artificial stimuli such as heat, cold, friction (i.e. massage by hand manipulation or forceful water), electricity, ultrasound, chemical reactions, or injury to the muscle tissue can also activate them.

Skeletal muscle contracts and relaxes relatively quickly. Visceral (smooth) muscle, which lines organs and blood vessels, contracts and relaxes more slowly and can maintain a state of contraction for longer periods of time. Stimulation of visceral muscle from nerve impulses causes a "squeezing" effect on organs creating movements such as constricting blood vessels or forcing food through the digestive system. Visceral and cardiac muscles are self-exciting, meaning they can repeat rhythmic contractions again and again without additional stimulus. The application of heat or cold over an area of an organ or the heart can speed up or slow down the rate of its muscular contractions.

F. The Digestive System

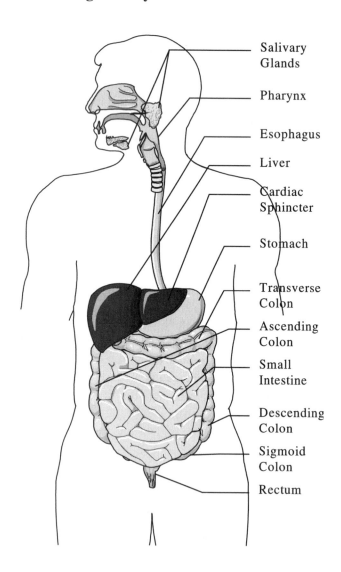

Salivary Glands

Pharynx

Esophagus

Liver

Cardiac Sphincter

Stomach

Transverse Colon

Ascending Colon

Small Intestine

Descending Colon

Sigmoid Colon

Rectum

The main organs of the digestive system are the mouth, pharynx, esophagus, stomach, small intestine, large intestine, and colon. This system functions to break down food, move the food products through each organ for absorption into the system, and eliminate unused portions. A muscular tube, known as the alimentary canal, extends from the mouth to the anus and is approximately 30 feet in length. Movement of food material through the digestive system is due to rhythmic waves of muscular contractions, known as peristalsis.

The mouth is the first part of the digestive system. It is used for receiving food and breaking the food into smaller particles to begin the digestive process. This is accomplished mechanically by chewing the food into smaller particles and chemically by mixing the food with saliva. Three pairs of salivary glands produce the mucous portion of saliva as well as an enzyme, known as salivary amylase, which begins the digestion of carbohydrates and starches. The food is then swallowed (deglutition) and passes through the pharynx (throat) into the esophagus.

The esophagus is the tubular portion of the digestive tract that begins at the bottom of the pharynx and leads to the stomach. It is a straight, collapsible tube approximately 10 inches long. The circular muscle fibers of the esophagus contract and squeeze the food downward into the stomach. There is a ring of muscle tissue between the esophagus and stomach which guards the opening of the esophagus and prevents food from re-entering the esophagus when the stomach contracts. This is known as the cardiac sphincter. (Sphincter meaning "ring-shaped" muscle.)

The stomach is a pouch-like organ located in the upper left portion of the abdominal cavity. Although its size varies, when it does not contain food it is about the size of a large sausage. The walls of the stomach bulge as it receives food from the esophagus. The stomach is divided into three regions: fundus, body, and pyloric. The fundic region is the first part of the stomach and acts as a temporary storage area. The body is the main, central part of the stomach, located between the fundic and pyloric sections. The pyloric region is the lowest section and becomes narrow as it approaches the small intestine. Glands located within the stomach secrete hydrochloric acid and pepsin, which further act on the food mixture to begin the digestion of proteins. The stomach functions to mix food matter with gastric juice, provide a small amount of absorption, begin the digestion of proteins, and move the food into the small intestine. The muscular sphincter located between the stomach and small intestine is the pyloric sphincter. This muscle protects the pyloric portion of the stomach so food material does not re-enter it as it is released into the small intestine.

The small intestine is the most important organ of absorption. It begins at the end of the stomach, continues to the opening of the large intestine, and is approximately 18 to 20 feet long. It is divided into three sections: the duodenum, the jejunum, and the ileum. The lining of the small intestine is covered with microvilli. These are tiny projections of epithelial and connective tissue that sweep the food material along and greatly increase the surface area of the small intestine for absorption. The small intestine also secretes several enzymes to complete the digestion of carbohydrates and proteins, and begin and end the breakdown and digestion of fats. All digestion is completed in the small intestine. At the end of the ileum, where it joins the large intestine, is the sphincter muscle called the Ileocecal valve. This muscle prevents the contents of the large intestine from backing up into the small intestine and generally remains closed unless the digestive process is taking place.

The large intestine is approximately 5 feet long, beginning in the lower right side of the abdominal cavity, crossing over to the left of the abdominal cavity, and moving downward to open to the outside of the body. The large intestine is divided into the cecum, which is the beginning, the colon, which is the main part, and the rectum. The inner lining of the large intestine is somewhat smooth; it does not contain microvilli like the small intestine since no digestion takes place. The large intestine receives food matter that could not be absorbed or digested by the body. The smooth muscles of the intestinal wall rhythmically contract and move this undigested matter along for final removal from the body through the rectum. Another main function of the large intestine is to reabsorb water and electrolytes (i.e. sodium, potassium, calcium, magnesium) so very little water or valuable electrolytes are lost in the feces. A large amount of bacteria normally reside in the large intestine. These bacteria can break down some substances, such as cellulose, which pass through the digestive system almost unchanged, and absorb them for use as an energy source. The action of the bacteria can also create certain vitamins to be absorbed by the intestinal wall and used to supplement the daily supply of dietary vitamins, such as Vitamin K and some of the B-complex vitamins. Once these vitamins are formed, they leave the large intestine and enter the blood.

Along with the main organs of digestion are organs which aide the digestive process. These are known as accessory organs of digestion and include the liver, pancreas, and gallbladder. The liver is located in the upper right region of the abdominal cavity and is the largest gland in the body. The liver is surrounded by a fibrous capsule and divided into many lobes (sections) by connective tissue. It is very vascular, containing a lot of blood vessels. The liver functions in the digestive process by producing bile, a liquid which causes large fat molecules to be broken down into smaller ones so they may be absorbed by the body in the small intestine. The liver produces about one pint of bile per day to aid in digestion. A large canal in the liver, known as the common bile duct, brings the bile to the duodenum of the small intestine. However, bile is first stored in the gallbladder, which is attached to the under surface of the liver. The gallbladder is a pear-shaped sac with a strong muscular layer in its walls. This organ stores bile between meals, and after stimulated to contract, moves the bile to the duodenum. The pancreas lies just behind the stomach. Most of the pancreas is made up of cells that produce pancreatic juice. The enzymes contained in pancreatic juice are able to digest carbohydrates, fats, and proteins. They contain sodium bicarbonate, which is used to neutralize the hydrochloric acid in the gastric juice from the stomach before it enters the small intestine. Pancreatic juice enters the duodenum of the small intestine at the same place as bile.

The temperatures of hot and cold influence both chemical and mechanical digestion as well as the physical properties of the muscle and connective tissues involved.

CHAPTER V SUMMARY - HUMAN ANATOMY AND PHYSIOLOGY

Anatomy: Branch of science that studies the form and structure of body parts.

Physiology: Branch of science that studies the function of the body and it's systems.

Circulatory System: Known as the cardiovascular system; consists of the heart and a closed system of blood vessels consisting of arteries, arterioles, capillaries, venules, veins, and the blood. Functions to transport oxygen, nutrients, and waste from body system to body system.

Heart: The heart is a four-chambered muscular pump.

Arteries: Arteries are strong, muscular, elastic blood vessels designed to carry blood away from the heart under high pressure.

Arterioles: Arterioles are small arteries that carry blood from the arteries to capillaries.

Capillaries: Capillaries are microscopic vessels, only one cell thick, capable of exchanging gases and nutrients between the blood and cells of the body.

Veins: Veins and smaller venules are composed primarily of connective and elastic tissue being less muscular than arteries. They contain one-way valves and function to carry blood toward the heart.

Pre-capillary Sphincter: A partial cuff of smooth muscle on the distal arteriole that controls blood flow to the capillaries by expanding and contracting.

Blood: Blood is the semi-liquid fluid, which courses through the circulatory system. It contains billions of formed (solid) elements known as blood cells in a liquid medium known as plasma. Of the total blood volume (near 5 liters in an adult) 55% is plasma; the remaining 45% is formed elements.

RBC's: Red blood cells or erythrocytes contain a substance known as hemoglobin, capable of combining with large quantities of oxygen and carbon dioxide. They are formed in red bone marrow and live about 120 days in circulation.

WBC's: White blood cells, or leukocytes, are fewer in number (but larger in size) than the RBC's. They are also formed by the red bone marrow but mature in different sites throughout the body, such as the liver, spleen and thymus. WBC's function is to guard against invasion of foreign organisms and chemicals and remove debris resulting from the death or injury of other cells. There are five major types of leukocytes (lymphocytes, monocytes, neutrophils, eosinophils, and basophils).

Motility: All WBC's are motile (they can move).

Diapedesis: Diapedesis is a process in which most types of WBC's move out of the capillaries into tissue by squeezing through the intercellular spaces of the capillary walls.

Chemotaxis: Chemotaxis is the name given to the chemical attraction of WBC's to an inflamed area.

Inflammation: The characteristics of inflammation include pain, heat, redness, and swelling. Redness and heat are explained by the increased blood flow. Swelling results from increased blood vessel permeability. The effects of kinins, prostaglandins and other neurotransmitters on nerve endings produce pain. Inflammation results when cells are damaged or destroyed.

Lymph: As plasma leaks from the blood capillaries and accumulates between tissue cells, it as known as interstitial fluid. Some of this fluid leaves the interstitial spaces through a series of lymphatic capillaries to become lymph.

Lymphatic System: The lymphatic system is closely related to the circulatory system. The lymphatic system contains microscopic capillaries, which are very permeable and a series of vein-like vessels that transport the lymph back to join the blood near the heart. Included in this system are a series of pea-sized filters known as lymph nodes. Specialized lymphatic capillaries called lacteals carry fats from the digestion system to the blood stream.

Nervous System: The nervous system consists of the brain, spinal cord and associated nerves. The brain and spinal cord comprise the Central Nervous System (CNS), which is completely encased within bony structures. The Peripheral Nervous System (PNS) is composed of nerves, which connect outlying parts of the body with the CNS. The nervous system functions to control and coordinate all body activities with rapid and precise action.

Neuron: The neuron consists of a main part called the cell body, one or more branch-like extensions known as dendrites, and one elongated projection known as an axon. Neurons are capable of communicating with other neurons and tissues. Nerves that carry nerve impulses from outer peripheral parts of the body into the brain or spinal cord are known as *sensory (afferent)* neurons. Nerves that carry messages out from the brain or spinal cord to parts of the body are known as *motor (efferent)* neurons.

Brain: The brain consists of the following four major divisions: cerebrum, cerebellum, diencephalon, and brain stem. The hypothalamus is the temperature-regulating center of the body.

Spinal Cord: The spinal cord is a slender nerve column, which extends downward from the brain stem through the vertebral canal to the bottom of the first lumbar vertebra. Spinal tracts transmit impulses that produce sensations of *crude touch, pain, temperature,* and *pressure;* and control many voluntary and involuntary movements.

Cranial Nerves: Twelve pairs of cranial nerves arise from various locations on the under surface of the brain and lead to parts of the head, neck, and trunk.

Spinal Nerves: There are thirty-one pairs of nerves, which arise from the spinal cord. These spinal nerves exit from the spinal cord and branch to form the many outlying nerves of the trunk and limbs. They conduct impulses between the spinal cord and the parts of the body not supplied by cranial nerves.

Dermatome: The skin segment supplied by a single spinal nerve is called a dermatome. Dermatomes provide a "map" of specific nerve activity.

Somatic Nervous System: System whose (efferent) fibers carry impulses from the CNS to skeletal muscle.

Autonomic Nervous System: System whose (efferent) fibers carry impulses from the CNS to visceral (smooth) muscle, cardiac muscle, and glandular (secretory) tissue. Includes the Sympathetic and Parasympathetic divisions.

Specialized Receptors: **Thermal Receptors** for the perception of temperature.
Baroreceptors for measuring blood pressure.
Mechanoreceptors are located in integumentary tissue for registering pressure, crude touch, fine touch, and vibration
Chemoreceptors for measuring carbon dioxide, hormones, enzymes, proteins, blood glucose, amino acids, fats, etc.
Nociceptors located in various tissues to register pain.

Hyper-Stimulation Analgesia: Melzack and Wall first described this phenomenon in 1965 as the "Gate-Control Hypothesis." It states that competitive stimulation (tactile, thermal, chemical, or electrical) may depress the transmission or recognition of pain (noxious) signals.

Temperature: The application of heat or cold influences nerve conduction.

Muscular System:	Accounts for nearly half of the body's weight. Responsible for body movements, posture, and generating heat.
Muscle types:	Skeletal, Visceral (Smooth), and Cardiac.
Heat:	Nearly 60% of sugar and oxygen catabolised by muscle becomes heat.
Contraction:	Normal muscle contraction requires adequate motor neuron stimulation, Ca, glucose, and oxygen
Temperature:	The application of heat or cold influences the strength and endurance of muscular contraction, as well as the ability of the muscle to relax.
Endocrine System:	The endocrine system is composed of a series of glands, which include the pituitary, thyroid, parathyroid, adrenal, pineal, and thymus glands as well as the pancreas, ovaries, placenta, and testes. The term "endocrine" is used to describe ductless glands that secrete their substances called hormones directly into bloodstream. The endocrine glands function to control the rates of certain chemical reactions, aid in the transport of substances through cell membranes, regulate stress responses, play vital roles in cell growth, and help regulate water and electrolyte balance.
Pituitary:	The pituitary gland is directly influenced by the hypothalamus and in turn produces at least eight hormones.
Pineal:	The pineal gland is a small structure located deep within the brain and is attached directly to the thalamus. *Melatonin* is secreted by the pineal gland in response to light conditions outside the body.
Thyroid:	The thyroid gland is located just below the larynx in front of the trachea. The thyroid produces two hormones (T3 & T4) that have a direct effect on cellular metabolic rate.
Adrenal:	The adrenal glands, which are attached to the top of each kidney, produce a number of hormones. Epinephrine (adrenaline) and nor-epinephrine both exert an influence on the body that is similar (but longer lasting) to the sympathetic nervous system (Fight or Flight) response. Aldosterone is also produced by the adrenal glands and is involved in the regulation of fluid and electrolyte balance. Cortisol from the adrenal cortex suppresses the immune response, and inflammation, while increasing blood sugar levels.

Prostaglandins: Prostaglandins (also known as tissue hormones) are chemical compounds formed in specialized cells of many tissues such as the heart, blood vessels, skin, and bronchi. These chemicals do not enter the blood stream, as do other hormones, but move by diffusion to influence nearby tissues. Prostaglandins are thought to aid in the control of such functions as respiration, vasodilation, inflammation, and cardiac rhythm.

Temperature: The application of heat or cold influences hormone production, transportation, and action at the target tissue site.

Integu-mentary System: The integumentary system is a complex sheet-like structure composed of the skin and its appendages. It comprises nearly 20 square feet of surface area, and it varies in thickness from 1/50th to 1/8th of an inch. It is in fact the largest organ of the body. The functions of the integument include protection, sensation, chemical production, and heat regulation.

Epidermis: The epidermis is less than 1/200th of an inch thick in most areas (the palms of the hands and soles of the feet are thicker). This layer of skin is composed of dead cells, which have been converted to the waterproof and chemical resistant protein substance, keratin, and millions of closely packed living cells.

Dermis: The deeper and thicker dermis is composed primarily of fibrous connective tissue - tough collagen fibers, elastin fibers, and a gel-like ground substance. The dermis contains an abundant supply of blood vessels (capillaries) and nerve endings. Also contained in the dermis are sweat glands, sebaceous glands, hair follicles, and small muscles called the arrector pili. On the average, each square inch of skin contains over 500 sweat glands, 1,000 nerve endings, yards of capillaries, over a 100 sebaceous glands, and hundreds of sensors (for pressure, heat, cold and pain).

Sub-Cutaneous Tissue: The subcutaneous tissue area contains both fibrous connective tissues (fascia) and adipose (fat). The adipose tissue of the subcutaneous layer serves as insulation, thus excluding heat from the outside and conserving interior heat. It also allows skin considerable freedom of movement. Superficial fascia (subcutaneous tissue) is most distinct over the abdomen and is thinnest on the dorsal surfaces of the hands and feet. Fibrous connective tissue (yellow) of the hypodermis is primarily composed of elastin fibers, differing from the deep fascia, which is composed primarily of collagen fibers (white fibrous connective tissue).

Temperature: The application of heat or cold influences skin function and physical properties of subcutaneous tissues.

52

Digestive System: A muscular tube, aka the alimentary canal, extends from the mouth to the anus and is approximately 30 feet in length. The system functions to chemically and mechanically break down food into microscopic elements for absorption and to eliminate unused portions.

Organs: The main organs of the digestive system are the mouth, pharynx, esophagus, stomach, small intestine, large intestine, and colon.

Accessory organs of digestion include the salivary glands, liver, pancreas, and gallbladder.

Temperature: Heat and cold influence both chemical and mechanical digestion, as well as the physical properties of both the muscle and connective tissues involved.

VI. TEMPERATURE REGULATION

A. Introduction

The body's temperature is regulated by behavioral regulation involving willed use of whatever means is available (exercise, clothing, meditation etc.) or by physiological regulation involving involuntary responses of the body (metabolism, circulatory changes, etc.). The body's core temperature (deep within the trunk) remains almost constant, except for the daily change (diurnal) in temperature or *circadian rhythm*--being controlled by the body's "internal clock" and "thermostat." The lowest temperature is in the early morning (3am -5am) and the highest temperature is in the late afternoon (4pm - 6pm). Normal core temperature is 98.6 degrees Fahrenheit (or 37 degrees Celsius). Diurnal changes, changes in exercise or food intake, sex, and age all affect the body's temperature. Older people may have a cooler core temperature. The temperature of visceral organs at the center of the body can be higher than the oral temperature. The temperature of muscles is usually lower than the core temperature, except when exercising. Temperature changes outside this range indicate disease or exposure to other influential conditions.

Different layers of the body have different temperatures. The depth of the tissue usually determines the temperature, and these variations are described as isotherm layers. The center of the body is the warmest. The ideal difference between the ambient temperature and the shell temperature of the body is 7 degrees F. Any greater difference becomes uncomfortable and changes begin to occur to compensate for this difference. A nude person could be exposed to a range of temperature from 55 degrees F to 140 degrees F in dry air while maintaining an almost constant internal body temperature.

LOCAL TISSUE TEMPERATURES

Location	Temperature	Location	Temperature
Tip of ear	83.64	Cheek	93.92
Breast	88	Pectoral area	94.5
Back of hand	90.5-91.76	Closed palm	94.64-96.18
Calf	92.5	Rectum	100
Forehead	93.38-93.92	Blood	102 average
Upper thigh	93.6	Brain	104
Forearm	93.7	Right ventricle	106
Open palm	93.9-94.6	Liver	106.5
Sternum	93.9	Left ventricle	107
Right Iliac fossa	93.9		

B. Mechanisms of Regulation

The body responds to external influences (applications of heat and cold) to protect tissues from damage and to maintain a constant core temperature. The CNS controls local and systemic responses to heat or cold. Information received from the sensory receptors (free nerve endings that respond to warm, cold, and thermal pain) located in the skin and probably in some deep body sites, transmit information through their afferent pathways to the hypothalamus and brain cortex. The inputs from the peripheral sensory receptors are a safety mechanism that protects the body against tissue damage.

Heat production is increased by the hypothalamus stimulating shivering by increasing the tone of skeletal muscle throughout the body. This increase in muscle metabolism increases the rate of heat production, often raising the total body heat production 50% before shivering occurs. When the tone of the muscles reaches a certain point, shivering occurs. This response is a result of feedback from the muscle spindle stretch reflex mechanism. Intense shivering can raise body heat production five times that of normal. Sympathetic stimulation or circulating norepinephrine and epinephrine in the blood causes an immediate increase in the rate of cellular metabolism. The hypothalamus increases the production of thyrotropin-releasing factor. This hormone stimulates secretion of thyrotropin, which in turn stimulates increased thyroxine output by the thyroid gland. Increased thyroxine increases the rate of cellular metabolism.

The cortex controls conscious awareness of these sensations. The body attempts to maintain an internal temperature of about 98.6 degrees F and a mean skin temperature of about 91.4 to 94 degrees F. When the internal or skin temperature changes, the thermoregulatory centers initiate responses to reestablish "the norm." Sweat glands are stimulated to cause heat loss by evaporation. The sympathetic centers of the hypothalamus are also stimulated, causing vasodilatation, increasing loss of heat from the skin. Evaporation always involves heat loss. When water evaporates from the body surface, 0.58 calories of heat are lost for each gram of water that evaporates. Insensible evaporation from the skin and lungs occurs at a daily rate of about 600 ml. as a result of diffusion of water molecules through the skin and respiratory surfaces, regardless of the temperature. However, regulating the rate of sweating can control evaporative loss of heat. Rapid evaporative cooling occurs when large quantities of sweat are secreted on the surface of the skin by the sweat glands. Sweat brings a large amount of heat to the surface. At ordinary room temperatures, evaporation accounts for approximately 25% of heat loss from the body.

The **precapillary sphincter** is a most significant anatomical structure with regards to hydrotherapy. This structure is a thickening of the muscular wall of the arteriole just before the capillaries. It responds to temperature changes, hormones, mechanical stimuli such as percussion, other massage strokes, and drugs. The precapillary sphincter's function is to control the blood flow to the capillaries and the blood pressure in the arteries.

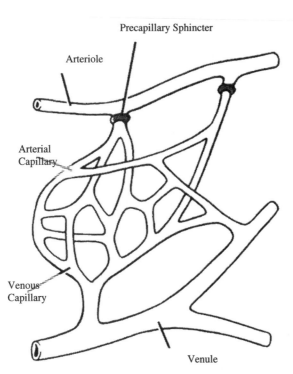

Precapillary Sphincter

Arteriole

Arterial Capillary

Venous Capillary

Venule

When cold is applied, vasoconstriction in the vessels of the peripheral tissue reduces the flow of blood to the skin and peripheral. This blood is diverted to viscera, and the central blood volume increases (**cold dieresis**). Mean body temperature decreases even though rectal temperature remains about the same. Cold exposure causes shivering to stimulate an increase in heat production. Muscles attached to the axial skeleton are involved, keeping heat in the core (for example teeth chattering). When exposed to cold, vasoconstriction can almost shut off the flow of blood to the surface skin and extremities. Any heat loss is then restricted to loss by conduction through muscle and fat, which are good insulators.

When heat is applied, vasoconstriction is released rapidly, and warm blood from the core will flow to the cold tissues. The core body temperature will decrease. Vasomotor changes easily control heat loss and keep heat production in balance. During exercise, muscles become the primary source of heat. The metabolic rate depends on the kind of exercise, the person's age, weight, and sex. During exercise, vasodilatation in the skin can increase heat flow tenfold, resulting in effective heat transfer from the body core to the skin. Until sweating occurs, increases in the blood flow to the skin can raise the skin temperature and heat loss occurs by convection and radiation. There are approximately 2,500,000 sweat glands in an adult male. Once sweating occurs, there is little change in skin temperature because the increased blood flow is accompanied by an increased sweat rate, resulting in removal of heat by evaporation. The maximum daily sweat rate is 10-15 liters.

CHAPTER VI SUMMARY - TEMPERATURE REGULATION

Body
Temperature: The body's core temperature remains almost constant, except for the daily change (diurnal) in temperature or circadian rhythm--being controlled by the body's "internal clock" and "thermostat." The lowest temperature is typically in the early morning (3am -5am) and the highest temperature is in the late afternoon (4pm - 6pm).

Normal Temps:		
Axillary	97.6 F	
Oral	98.6 F (37 C)	
Rectal	99.6 F	

Warmest Body Areas:				
Left ventricle	107 F	Brain	104 F
Liver	106.5 F	Blood	102 F average
Right ventricle	106 F		

Coolest Body Areas:				
Open palm	93.9-94.6 F	Breast	88 F
Forehead	93.38-93.92 F	Tip of ear	83.64 F
Back of hand	90.5-91.76 F		

Regulation: The body responds to external influences (applications of heat and cold) to protect tissues from damage and to maintain a constant core temperature.

Heat
Conservation: Vasoconstriction in the vessels of the peripheral tissue reduces the flow of blood to the skin and peripheral structures, thus limiting heat loss by convection and radiation.

Heat Gain: CNS based controls cause more heat to be created via the pituitary (TSH) and thyroid (T3 & T4) glands to increase (primarily muscle) metabolism and therefore, the production of heat.

Heat Loss: Excess heat is carried to the surface of the body by the blood to be disposed. The primary methods of heat loss include increased superficial circulation via the relaxation of the precapillary sphincters, increased passive evaporation, increased radiation and convection via increases in blood perfusion, and finally, increased active evaporation via sweating.

The precapillary sphincter responds to temperature changes, hormones, mechanical stimuli such as percussion, other massage strokes, drugs, and functions to control the blood flow to the capillaries.

VII. PHYSIOLOGICAL EFFECTS OF HYDROTHERAPY

A. Introduction

Hydrotherapy treatments require an understanding of the physiological responses resulting from the application of heat or cold. The effects on body tissues and the functions of the body systems are numerous and varied. For example, heat may be indicated for a chronic ankle sprain. However, if this patient also had diabetes and poor circulation, heat would be contraindicated because the vascular system might not be able to handle the removal of the excessive heat or metabolic wastes. The amount of surface area involved determines the result; the larger the surface area involved the greater the effect. The physiological effects of hydrotherapy are categorized as being mechanical, chemical, or thermal.

1. **Mechanical** effects are produced by the impact of water on the body by whirlpools, sprays, douches, and frictions.

2. **Chemical** effects are produced when water is taken by mouth or used an irrigation of a body cavity.

3. **Thermal** effects are produced by the application of water at temperatures above or below that of the body. The greater the difference (gradient) in temperature between the skin and environment, the greater the effect. Thermal effects are by far the most important in hydrotherapy.

The results of heat and cold applications are further classified as **local, systemic,** and **reflex**. The body's response to these applications produces certain physiological changes, depending on the **temperature difference, length of application,** and **amount of body surface involved**. These changes generally include either safety mechanisms to prevent tissue damage or attempts to maintain an internal (core) temperature of about 98.6 degrees F.

Extreme temperatures, below freezing and above 113 degrees F, can injure human tissue. Our body can tolerate a temperature range of about 50 degrees F. Pain is perceived when the temperature rises toward 109 degrees F or when it falls below 59 degrees F. Pain is a warning that the tissue can be damaged. A nude person could be exposed to a range of temperature from 55 degrees F to 140 degrees F in dry air and maintain an almost constant internal body temperature.

The following chart defines a full range of temperature possibilities for hydrotherapy and the response of the body to these temperature ranges:

Description	Range Degrees in F	Comments
Dangerously hot	125	Can injure tissue
Painfully hot	111-124	Intolerable
Very hot	105-110	Can tolerate for short period of time
Hot*	100-104	Tolerable but skin turns red
Warm	92-100	Comfortable
Neutral	94-97	Average skin temperature
Tepid	80-92	Slightly below skin temperature
Cool	70-80	Produces goose flesh
Cold*	55-70	Tolerable but uncomfortable
Very cold	32-55	Painfully cold

*Hot and cold temperatures as would be normally used in hydrotherapy

B. Effects

Generally speaking, **local** effects are immediate responses and occur in the area being treated. Sometimes called thermal shock reactions, they are reactions to thermal sensory experiences (heat or cold applications). Depending on the temperature of the application local changes include: vasodilation or vasoconstriction, increased or decreased circulation, increased or decreased rate of blood flow, increased or decreased metabolism in tissue, muscle relaxation, and an analgesic effect.

Systemic effects are changes that occur in the functionally related group of parts or organs as a result of the treatment not being limited to the area of application. Again, depending on the temperature of the application, these effects include: changes in internal temperature, general changes in vasomotor and sudomotor (sweat control) response, cardiovascular responses which include generalized changes in vasodilation of cutaneous vessels, peripheral blood pressure and blood flow, changes in heart and respiration, changes in metabolic activity, and changes in nerve activity and renal responses.

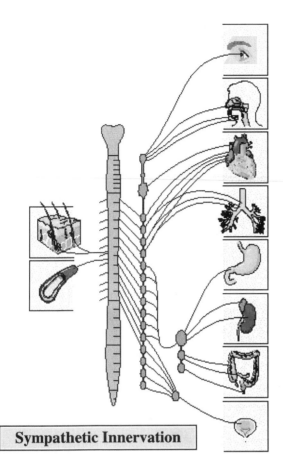

Sympathetic Innervation

Reflex effects are not the immediate responses of the skin area, but effects that occur elsewhere in the body and which are mediated by the Autonomic Nervous System. A reflex arc is set up from the afferent nerve fibers of the skin surface, which carry the stimulus to the spinal cord. This stimulus is then communicated to an efferent autonomic fiber that communicates to an autonomic ganglion, which in turn sends this stimulus on to the organ supplied or another predictable destination. In other words, reflex effects may be repeated in a predictable fashion. These effects produce changes in vasomotor or circulatory activity, visceromotor or musculature, and secretory or glandular tissue. The reflex effects are based anatomically on the segmental relationships of the skin and major organs.

The following chart shows the relationship of internal structures and spinal nerves:

Organ	Segment of Spinal Cord Innervation
Heart & aorta	Thoracic 1-4
Lungs	Thoracic 1-7 (commonly 2-5)
Stomach	Thoracic 7-9
Intestines	Thoracic 9-11
Liver & gall bladder	Thoracic 3, 6-9
Kidneys	Thoracic 10 to Lumbar 1
Testes	Thoracic 10
Bladder Mucosa	Sacral 3-4
Bladder Muscle	Thoracic 11 to Lumbar 1
Uterus, upper part	Thoracic 11, 12
Uterus, lower part	Sacral 3, 4

C. Manipulation of Blood Flow

Hydrotherapy may be used to manipulate blood flow. This result is accomplished by several methods, summarized as follows:

1. The principles of **derivation** (the drawing of blood or lymph from one part of the body by increasing the amount of blood or lymph moving *to* another part) and **retrostasis** (the driving of blood or lymph *from* one area of the body to another area) make use of the circulatory effects of heat and cold. Heat produces derivation, blood flows toward heat; cold produces retrostasis, blood flows away from cold. In the case of a congestive headache, heat applied to the feet draws blood and lymph to the feet and away from the head, reducing congestion in the painful area. An ice bag to the head would drive blood and lymph from the congested head to the lower parts of the body. The most effective and optimum treatment combines both applications.

2. **Revulsive** effects involve a single prolonged application of heat followed by a single brief application of cold. The application of heat intensifies the latter application of cold, which moves blood away from the local area. This is a very powerful local treatment for moving blood.

3. **Collateral circulation** involves the principles of both derivation and retrostasis but in a much more restricted area. In collateral circulation, blood flow modifications in a *superficial* artery are used to change the circulation of a *deep* artery from the same trunk. For example, when an arterial trunk bifurcates into superficial and deep branches (and the circulation is normal), blood flow through the two branches is about equal. When cold is applied over the start of the superficial branch, that branch constricts, causing decreased blood flow. At the same time the deep branch dilates, increasing blood flow. This is a retrostatic reaction. If hot were applied to the superficial branches, the results are opposite. For example, the radial and ulnar arteries split off from the brachial artery. The radial artery is superficial and the ulnar artery is deep. These applications would influence the radial artery directly and the ulnar artery indirectly.

4. The **arterial trunk reflex** is based on the principle that whatever influences an arterial trunk will also influence the smaller vessels fed by that trunk. When hot is applied to an arterial trunk, it dilates, carrying more blood--but so do the distal arteries branching off from the trunk. This is an important principle in treating diabetic patients with circulatory problems. A small hot application over the femoral artery causes dilation in the anterior tibial artery. The circulation is increased in the compromised area without raising the local metabolic rate to dangerous levels.

5. The **spinal cord reflex** is based on the principle that each vital center has a corresponding area of skin, which is reflexively connected to it. For example, a long cold application to the skin over the spleen would constrict the skin vessels overlying the spleen, as well as constrict the splenic vessels. Also the left hand is reflexively

related to the right hand and vice versa, as well as the shoulders. This principle can be used to help the healing of a broken arm. Hydrotherapy techniques cannot be applied to the arm in the cast but can be to the other arm.

As one can see, some of these methods could result in conflicting results. Here are some general guidelines:

1. Smaller areas of application elicit more reflexive effects than direct (an ice bag to the inside of the thighs will constrict the uterine vessels).
2. Larger areas of application elicit more direct effects than reflexive (a hot full-body bath has minimal effects on reflex points).
3. Greater intensity treatments elicit more reflexive effects (a very cold application to the hand gives stronger direct and reflexive effects to the brain, whereas a more neutral application would have predominantly more direct effects).
4. The closer the area treated to the reflex organ the more reflexive the effect (applications over the head or heart tend to be reflexive, but a hot foot bath has a stronger derivative effect because of the greater distance between the feet and the brain, lungs, and bladder).

There are variables, which come into play when using hydrotherapy to manipulate blood flow. As an example, the methods of manipulation of the blood flow and the varying applications in applying hot and cold in treating *"cerebral congestion"* and *"congestive headache" or "vascular headache"* are discussed as follows:

1. Direct Method - Cold to the head (cold is depressive).
2. Revulsive Method - Hot application followed by Cold to head (cold vasoconstricts and moves blood away).
3. Derivative/Retrostatic Method - Hot to the feet & Cold to the head (Hot draws blood to feet and cold pushes blood away from the head).
4. Collateral Method - Hot to face over maxillary artery (diverts blood from deeper branches of artery).
5. Arterial trunk Method - Ice pack to the carotids (contracts smaller vessels).
6. Spinal cord reflex Method - Cold to the palms of the hands (moves blood from head via reflex association with that area).

In hydrotherapy the **hydrostatic effect** is the shifting of fluid from one part of the body to another. When a large area of the body is exposed to heat, blood vessels in the skin dilate and large quantities of blood shift from the interior to the skin's surface. Conversely, when cold is applied in the same manner, the blood shifts to the interior from the limbs. Clinically, this principle is used in treating congestive headaches, congested nose and sinuses, and pulmonary congestion in the early stages of pneumonia. Derivation by dilatation of the blood vessels of the skin is often effective in relieving these congested conditions.

D. Effects of Heat

l. Introduction

Depending on the intensity of the heat application, the immediate reaction a person may experience is as follows: mild application produces an analgesic effect; moderate application produces a stimulating affect; extreme application produces fear or pain. These sensations are called thermal shock reactions resulting from the sensory experience of the thermal application. Other responses include local sweating and erythema.

It is generally accepted that heat produces the following therapeutic effects:

1. Initially excitatory and later depressant/sedative to nervous system
2. The extensibility of collagen tissue is increased.
3. The fluidity of connective tissue matrix is increased.
4. Joint stiffness is decreased and range of motion increased.
5. Pain is relieved.
6. Muscle spasms are reduced or relieved.
7. Inflammatory products are removed and edema may be reduced.
8. Blood flow is increased.

2. Local Effects

Skin and subcutaneous fat are poor thermal conductors. They retain a large amount of heat and conduct little heat to deeper tissues. Superficial heat modalities do not elevate the temperature of deep musculature or increase blood flow; deep heat modalities (diathermy, ultrasound, etc.) are capable of increasing blood flow and temperature to the deeper structures. Studies show that a long, intense application of moist heat penetrates about 3.4 centimeters, reaching the superficial layers of muscle. The local effects of heat are largely confined to the skin and subcutaneous tissues where certain physiological changes take place. These changes are discussed as they relate to the rise in local tissue temperature.

 The metabolic rate of cellular activity increases. The chemical effects of metabolites will aid in vasodilation, which cause changes to the blood cells. The numbers of WBCs are increased as well as movement. Van Hoff's Law states that the speed of chemical reactions increases two to three times for each rise in l0 degrees C. The increase in the metabolic rate increases the activity of leukocytes and phagocytosis, facilitating the healing process, and repairing tissue damage. Because of this fact and the increased local circulation, heat applications may be indicated to hasten the healing of damaged tissues and clear the interstitial tissues of inflammatory by-products, hemorrhage, or edema. The number of leukocytes increases because they migrate through the vessel walls in heated areas. Diaphoresis (sweating) results in increased white blood cells and increased circulation. Local blood alkaline levels decrease with applied heat. Leukocytes are also more effective in fighting bacteria because of the increase in heat and decrease in pH level. White blood cells are the major component of the immune system. The body has 300 trillion WBCs available to fight and protect the body from foreign invaders. There are approximately 60 trillion (20%) WBCs circulating in the blood stream during normal conditions. Hot (as well as cold) stimulate the number of circulating white blood cells and their intensity. If any of the vascular, renal or sweat balance mechanisms of the body are compromised, the pH balance may be upset and unfavorable reactions may occur.

Vascular changes occur as a result of vasodilation. The application of local heat increases the flow of blood to the skin. Much of the heat is dissipated by the blood flow and this protects the skin from injury. Vasodilation causes localized redness (erythema). It is thought that the increased sweating releases Bradykinin, which in turn causes the erythema. Vasodilation is also thought to be produced by local axon reflexes initiated by the stimulation of skin receptors. The vasodilation results in: (1) an increase in nutrients and leukocytes which aid in tissue healing, (2) an increase in the removal of metabolites, decreasing pain or muscle spasms caused by an accumulation of these products, and (3) an increase in the amount of cooler blood arriving in the area and removal of warmer blood, helping to prevent tissue damage from excessive heating. When blood flow is increased to an area, the blood vessels dilate while the remainder of the vessels in the area contract, decreasing the blood pressure in that area. This vasodilation explains why heat applied to an arthritic joint or congested nerve/muscle reduces the pain. As the blood vessels in the inflamed area contract, tension is relieved and pain is reduced; when using heat, several conditions may present special considerations. For example, patients with edema or local bleeding should receive only mild heat, if any. The integrity of the vessels is important. With arteriosclerosis, the arterial wall may be compromised, limiting dilatation. These vessels may not be able to handle the increased blood flow. Contraindications and precautions are discussed as they apply to each treatment in Chapter VII, Therapeutic Techniques and Procedures.

3. Systemic Effects

Systemic changes occur that are not local reactions but affect the entire body. Cardiovascular responses include generalized vasodilation of cutaneous vessels, drop in peripheral blood pressure (there is increased pressure in both the arterial and venous capillaries), and increased heart and pulse rate. Studies have shown that when wet heat is applied to the forearm for 20-30 minutes at 113 degrees F, the rate of blood flow was doubled and lasted for approximately one hour after the application was removed. There was also an increase in the oxygen content of the blood. Blood volume is increased because there is a shift of fluid from the tissues to the blood stream. As previously discussed, only mild heat, if any, should be used if edema or bleeding is present. After an acute injury, heat should not be applied for approximately 72 hours. Rest, ice, compression and elevation (RICE) should be used during the first 72 hours. The health of the vessels must be considered. If local heat is applied and the increased blood flow cannot be handled, tissue damage, ischemia, or necrosis may occur. The body's responses may fluctuate when attempting to regulate body temperature. For example, when the heart rate increases there may be an increase in blood pressure. Conversely, when the heart rate drops, there may be a decrease in blood pressure. If it drops too low, the heart will then increase its rate again. Eventually the blood pressure will stabilize, with only a slight increase in heart rate. A drop in blood pressure, reducing the blood flow to the brain, may cause fainting. It is not uncommon for debilitated people to faint as they experience the systemic responses to a rise in temperature. Systemic vascular shunting may occur when the internal temperature is high. In an effort to cool the body, blood may be shunted from deep circulatory systems to peripheral systems. This volume of blood gives off more heat. This reduction in blood flow from the deep systems is only temporary or serious damage could occur to the organs.

Respiratory changes occur. The warm air given off by breathing helps the body to remove some heat. Because the air is moist, evaporation of the moisture in the air and mucous membranes helps the body cool. "Panting" is not a normal response to heat in humans, as it is in animals. In humans, this is a sign of metabolic acidosis and is a signal to discontinue the heat treatment or exercise.

The integumentary system is also affected. Sweating increases during this time and heat is dissipated through evaporation. The eccrine sweat glands stimulate sweating when the skin temperature rises above approximately 91.4 degrees and with almost any rise in core temperature. Most of the eccrine glands are thermoregulatory. Sweat cools the skin surface by: (1) bringing heat to the surface in the fluid, (2) evaporation of the fluid on the skin when exposed to air, using calories of heat to vaporize the sweat and cool the surface and, (3) transferring heat from the sweat on the skin to adjacent cooler air molecules (convection). Profuse sweating may result in loss of water, salt and small amounts of urea, uric acid, creatinine, phosphates, sulfates, and lactic acid.

The muscular system is affected. If limited range of motion or nerve compression is due to shortened collagen tissues, heat is of great value. Collagen tissue can be extended when heated, as well as joint capsules, scare tissue and tendons. The viscoelastic properties and collagen organizational arrangement change when heat is applied, allowing for this elongation by stretching. Studies have shown that heat results in greater inhibitory impulses from the Golgi tendon organs, allowing a reduction in muscle spasm and relaxation.

Skeletal changes occur. The joints move more freely when heated. When the skin is heated to 113 degrees F, the underlying joint moves about 20% more freely. This change is thought to be produced by the reduction in tension of soft tissue and non-elastic tissues.

There are also changes in the nervous system. Motor functions of the nervous system control contraction of skeletal muscles, contraction of smooth muscle in internal organs and secretions. A local analgesic effect occurs with the application of heat. The pain and temperature pathways are close together in long spinal tracts. Heat competes with the pain impulses, overriding them, and producing this analgesic effect.

Urine excretion (diuresis) increases because of the increase in alkalinity and excretions by the kidneys, helping the body rid itself of metabolic by-products. Patients with renal disease or urine retention problems should not be exposed to frequent or prolonged heat treatments.

4. Reflex Effects

Applications of hot (or cold) not only affect the skin, but also reflexively affect other body parts through the nervous system. The afferent nerve fibers from the skin surface carry stimulus to the spinal cord through the posterior nerve root. The stimulus synapses with efferent nerve fibers, which carry the stimulus from the anterior spinal nerve root to an autonomic ganglion, which passes through another synapse and travels to the organ supplied. Reflex heating refers to the fact that an application of heat to one area of the body can result in an increase in cutaneous circulation and other reactions in another area. These changes occur almost immediately. This technique is also called consensual or remote heating. There is a segmental relationship between the skin and organs. Studies as early as the late 19th century concluded that pain impulses from diseased organs produced pain in the skin area receiving sensory innervation from the same segment of the spinal cord. Cutaneous stimulation elicits reflex visceral reactions (especially vasomotor changes and changes in tonic state of visceral musculature). Therefore, visceral conditions can be influenced by stimulation of a corresponding cutaneous area. In cases where heating an area can cause tissue damage due to pathological conditions, heating the reflexive part can increase circulation to the compromised area.

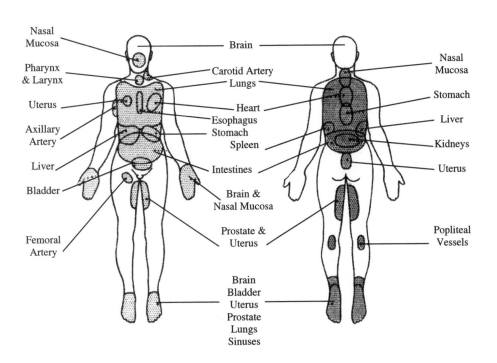

Local Reflex Skin Areas & Associated Structures

Reflex Effects of **Prolonged Heat** application are summarized as follows:

Location of Application	Reflex Effect
One extremity	Vasodilatation in contralateral extremity.
Abdominal Wall	Decreased intestinal blood, intestinal mobility, and secretion of stomach acid.
Pelvic Area	Relaxation in pelvic organ musculature, blood vessels are dilated, and menstrual flow increased.
Heart Region	Increased heart rate, lower blood pressure, and force.
Chest Area	Promotes ease of respiration, and expectoration.
Kidney area (anterior & posterior)	Moist heat increases urine production.

E. Effects of Cold

l. Introduction

Although you might think that the body's reaction to the application of cold is just the opposite of heat, there are some differences. Usually the metabolic responses are the opposite, but the vascular responses are not. Variables for cold modalities include the temperature, the difference between the skin and the modality temperature, the duration of the application, the vascular supply to the area, and the thermal conductivity and thickness of the tissue layers. The thermal shock reactions are very similar to those of heat, depending on the degree of the cold application, ranging from an analgesic effect, to fear, or pain.

The temperature of the cold modality is very important. The colder the modality, the greater danger of tissue damage. However, the greater the difference between the temperature of the modality and the skin, the greater the effect. Careful consideration and review of the critical cold temperatures is important before using a super cooling modality.   Cold must be used carefully to bring about the desired physiological changes, without injuring tissue or causing the "fight or flight" response.

2. Local Effects

The local effects and immediate responses to cold are local vasoconstriction with blanching of the skin and local piloerection. The blood flow is restricted, causing a slowing of local circulation, and local tissue temperature is reduced. Some believe that cold inhibits the release of histamines resulting in blanching. The initial vasoconstriction response lasts approximately 10-30 minutes. The viscosity of the blood increases slightly. Because of the decrease in venous flow to the area, there can be an increase in the content of carbon dioxide in the blood, accounting for the blue color of cooled skin. The prolonged cold application acts as a depressant or sedative, lowering the temperature and lessening vital activity. A short-cold application is an excitant, it is very stimulating, and reduces fatigue. It causes contraction of the small vessels in the skin and internal organs, quickly followed by dilatation.

The integumentary system is affected in several ways. Perspiration is diminished at first, with a subsequent increase. The smaller arteries, veins, and capillaries of the skin will spasm, causing pallor; but later, flush occurs from active dilatation of the vessels. The muscular and connective tissues of the skin contract. Prolonged applications lessen the skin's sensibility and diminish reflex effects. Smooth muscular fibers of the skin, blood vessels, bladder, bowels, etc. are excited.

The metabolic rate also decreases, which can slow the healing process. Post-traumatic edema can be reduced by using cooling modalities. However, there are mixed reports. Some studies have shown that the edema is increased or returns as the tissue warms. Inflammation caused by histamine and serotonin could be inhibited by the use of cold. However, inflammation initiated by prostaglandins could be aggravated by cold. Therefore, it is important for the therapist to remain current on research. In recent studies, the use of hot, cold, and/or contrast modalities has had mixed results. The studies also have mixed results with regard to the response of certain inflammatory conditions, depending on what chemical mediators produced the inflammation.

3. Systemic Effects

As the temperature lowers, the sensory and motor peripheral nerves are affected by cooling when firing of all pain and tactile neurons decreases. The excitation and nerve conduction velocity of neurons decrease relative to the temperature. The sensations felt during the use of a cold modality might first be cold, then painfully cold, then less cold, and more pain sometimes perceived as warmth or burning. However, numbness and anesthesia eventually occur. Ice massage often elicits this type of response in patients. Cold affects deeper tissues than does heat. This result is due to the fact that there is a greater difference in temperature gradient between the modality and the skin. Also, heat is not convected from the area as rapidly. The thickness of the subcutaneous fat layer, as well as the vascular status in the area, affects the results of the cold treatment. In areas where the vascular supply is poor, cooling is enhanced, and this can be dangerous. There are secondary vascular responses that occur to protect tissue. If the duration or intensity of the cold application is significant, tissue damage can occur. However, if the vascular tissue is healthy, after about 15-30 minutes, blood flow increases to the tissue in danger of being damaged. Cold applications decrease spasticity caused by motor neuron lesions. This is especially beneficial to multiple sclerosis patients. It is thought that the cold reduces the local motor excitability by acting as an anesthesia on peripheral sensory end organs, which inhibits the nerve activity.

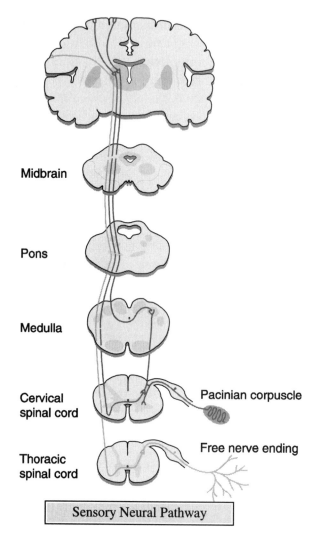

Midbrain

Pons

Medulla

Cervical
spinal cord

Thoracic
spinal cord

Pacinian corpuscle

Free nerve ending

Sensory Neural Pathway

Respiration is then increased because carbon dioxide levels increase. Muscular irritability and energy decreases with prolonged cold applications.

4. Reflex Effects

Reflex Effects of **Prolonged Cold** applications are summarized as follows:

Location of Application	Reflex Effect
Trunk of Artery	Artery and branches contract.
Skin over Nose, back of Neck and Hands	Blood vessels of nasal mucosa contract.
Heart Region	Heart rate decreases/stroke volume increases (amount of blood pumped with each contraction).
Abdominal Skin	Increased intestinal blood flow, intestinal Motility, and acid secretion.
Pelvic Area (Sitz baths)	Stimulates muscles of the pelvic organs.
Thyroid Gland	Blood vessels contract and decrease in function.
Hands & Skin of Scalp	Contraction of blood vessels in brain.
Acutely Inflamed Joints & Bursae	Vasoconstriction, relief of pain, and hastens recovery.
Acute Trauma	Vasoconstriction and relief of pain, swelling, and hemorrhage in the area.

* Reflex responses to an application of cold also include an adaptive heating reaction with vasodilation (aka: hunting response), which represents an attempt by the organism to maintain homeostasis. This response generally occurs when the local skin temperature is less than 10° C (75.6° F) or during prolonged periods of cooling. The "hunting response" is thought to be a protective mechanism designed to prevent tissue damage from prolonged ischemia.

Reflex Effects of **Short Cold** applications are summarized as follows:

Location	Effect
Dilated vessels in skin	Intense cooling for 30 seconds increasing peripheral vasoconstriction.
Face, Hands & Head	Increased mental alertness and activity.
Heart region	Increased heart rate and stroke volume.
Reflex area of an organ	Intense, short application, such as with percussion douche, may increase the functional activity of the organ.
Chest	With the use of friction or percussion, initial increase in respiratory rate but later produces slower, deeper respiration.

Cold is very beneficial for "refrigeration" anesthesia before surgery for the amputation of a limb. There is a numbing or analgesic affect. It is also beneficial for acute pain of the joints, bursitis, sprains, and other local trauma. Applications of cold are very successful in treating burn victims; reducing pain and the amount of tissue damage, as well as reducing redness and blistering in less serious burns.

The general effects of cold are stimulating, after an initial depressant stage, and have a tonic reaction. Prolonged applications decrease metabolic activity. The heart initially beats faster then slower, vessels contract, nerves are numbed, respiration slows and deepens, and the stomach increases secretions and motility. Both the number of RBCs and WBCs are increased, as is phagocytosis, with short chilling.

F. Effects of Contrast Heat and Cold Applications

Reflex effects of contrast heat and cold procedures stimulate the related tissues and organs as in the contrast bath.

The local effects of contrast heat and cold treatments are stimulating and increase local circulation. A 30-minute contrast bath, immersing only the lower extremities, produces a 95% increase in local blood flow. When all four extremities are immersed simultaneously, there is an 100% increase in blood flow to the upper extremities and a 70% increase to the lower. The frequency and duration of the contrasting baths is open to debate. However, the cold immersion need only be long enough to produce vasoconstriction, and this occurs in less than a minute. Generally, the hot water immersion lasts four minutes and the cold water immersion less than a minute. The treatment is usually repeated for a total time of 30 minutes.

G. Comparison of Heat versus Cold Applications

The following charts summarize the physiological responses, the effects or results of these responses, and the clinical significance of local heat and/or cold applications for use in hydrotherapy.

Summary of Physiologic Responses to Applied HEAT		
Physiological Response	**Result**	**Clinical Significance**
Mild heat sensation	Analgesic/sedative	Decreases pain and spasms; aids relaxation.
Moderate heat sensation	Autonomic	Invigorating.
Extreme heat sensation	"Fight or flight" reaction	Pain/fear.
Changes in skin color	Erythema	Increased blood flow.
Increased metabolic rate	Increased healing & waste production	Increases heat production and tissue temperature.
Increased blood flow	Increased bleeding	Increased healing
Reflex response	Increased cutaneous blood flow in related areas of the body	Transitory effect.
Increased capillary permeability	Increase/decrease in interstitial fluid	Increase/decrease edema.
Increased sweating	Increased cooling	Decreases fluid/salt balance in body.
Fluctuation in cardiovascular activity	Changes in heart rate and blood pressure	Puts stress on CV system.
Increased respiration	Little value in maintaining thermal homeostasis	Indicates heat distress.
Decreased joint stiffness	Increase speed and freedom of joint movement	Increases agility.
Increased extensibility of non-elastic tissues	Assist in stretching tendons and scar tissue	Increases range of motion.
Increased peripheral nerve activity	Increased conduction velocity	Motor function increases

© Pine Island Publishers Inc. 2003

72

Summary of Physiological Responses to Applied COLD

Physiological Response	Result	Clinical Significance
Mild cold sensation	Analgesic/sedative	Decreases pain and spasms & relaxing.
Moderate cold sensation	Autonomic	Invigorating and stimulant.
Extreme cold sensation	"Fight or flight" reaction	Pain and fear.
Initial vasoconstriction (superficial)	Decreased superficial bleeding	May not alter or may increase deep blood flow.
Secondary vasofluctuations	Blood flow varies	Protects tissues from cold injury.
Change in skin color	Initial: blanching	Decrease in superficial blood flow.
	Secondary: redness	Increase in superficial blood flow.
Increased blood viscosity	Decreased blood flow.	Retards bleeding.
Decreased metabolic rate	Decreased inflammation; may decrease edema	May retard healing.
Rapid muscular contraction (shivering)	Increased metabolic rate	Maintaining thermal homeostasis.
Piloerection	Goose bumps	Ineffectual attempt to maintain homeostasis.
Decreased extensibility of nonelastic tissue	Decreased ability to stretch tendons and joint capsules	Decreased range of motion.
Decreased peripheral nerve activity	Decreased firing and conduction of motor and sensory nerves.	May decrease spasticity.
Possible decreased temperature of joint tissues and fluids	Increased joint stiffness and decreased activity of fluid enzymes.	Decreased speed of joint motion. May decrease destruction degenerative disease (Rheumatoid Arthritis)

H. Choice of Modality

There are many factors affecting the choice of a thermal modality. The timing of the application, its frequency, the hour of the day, the location of the application, the materials used, the wetness of the application; and the various techniques used, such as friction or pressure, all affect the outcome of the treatment. Always consult the patient's physician regarding any thermal treatments when there are exacerbating conditions. **Be cautious**. Discontinue treatment if the patient complains of or shows visible signs of discomfort, increased respiration, or pulse rate. Take the pulse before, during, and after prolonged or vigorous heat treatments. If the pulse rate of a young adult approaches double his/her resting rate, discontinue treatment. In other words, the pulse rate should not exceed (220 minus the patients age ÷2). Also, if the strength of the pulse diminishes or the blood pressure changes, treatment should be discontinued.

Other precautions that should be considered include:

1. Be sure the patient is properly hydrated before a prolonged heat treatment.
2. Fatigue is not conducive to thermal treatments.
3. Children and elderly patients may not react as expected.
4. Good physical condition enhances a treatment.
5. The patient should be comfortably warm before treatment.
6. Friction/percussion increases the reaction.
7. Eating just before or after treatment, as well as use of alcohol/drugs and sugar can decrease the results of treatment.
8. Certain conditions decrease the ability of some organs to handle the physiological changes that occur. Be aware and consult with the treating physician. Changes may have to be made to prevent negative reactions.

The following chart provides guidelines for selecting either a hot or cold modality for certain conditions. It is only a *guideline* and each patient is different.

Problem	Response Desired	Heat	Cold
Pain	Analgesia by hyperstimulation	Yes	Yes
	Anesthesia	No	Yes
Muscle spasms	Reduce pain by clearing metabolites	Yes	No
Upper motor neuron spasticity	Affects motor nerves	Yes- briefly	Yes - up to 90 min.

Problem	Response Desired	Heat	Cold
Bleeding or hemorrhage	Vasoconstriction	No	Yes - for 15-30 min.
Edema	Unclear evidence		
	Acute edema	No *	Yes
	Chronic edema	Yes *	No *
Wound healing	Increased blood flow/ metabolic activity	Yes	No
Frostbite	Hasten healing	Yes	No
Hypotension (from standing)	Vascular reaction	No	Yes
Joint stiffness	Increased mobility	Yes	No
Inability to perform skilled movements	Increased neuron firing and nerve conduction velocity	Yes	No
Arthritic joints (Osteoarthritis or non-acute rheumatoid)	Decreased pain/stiffness Increased use	Yes	No
Acute rheumatoid arthritis	Reduce enzyme activity in joint fluid/decrease pain	Superficial Yes	Yes
Shortness of soft tissue	Increased extensibility of non-elastic tissue	Yes	No
General stimulant or relaxation	Mild/moderate sensory stimulation	Yes	Yes
CNS Problems	Increased firing of sensory neurons	Yes, but cold is better	Yes

* Efficacy of either hot or cold applications is unsubstantiated

CHAPTER VII SUMMARY - PHYSIOLOGICAL EFFECTS OF HYDRO TX

Mechanical: Effects produced by the physical force or impact of water on the body by whirlpools, sprays, douches, and frictions.

Chemical: Effects produced when water is taken by mouth or used in irrigation of a body cavity, as with drinking a hypertonic laxative solution.

Thermal: Effects are produced by the application of water at temperatures above or below that of the body. The greater the difference (gradient) in temperature between the skin and environment, the greater the effect. Thermal effects are by far the most important in hydrotherapy.

Factors Influencing Effects:
1. Temperature difference between therapeutic application and body part
2. Length of time of therapeutic application
3. Amount of body surface exposed to therapeutic application

Effects of Heat:

1. Local: (effects are brief & superficial due to vasodilation)
   - Increased cellular metabolic rate
   - Increased vasodilation & diaphoresis
   - Increased vascular permeability
   - Increased blood flow to area
   - Erythema
   - Increased diapedesis
   - Increased leukocytosis (300 – 500%)
   - Increased chemotaxis
   - Increased phagocytosis
   - Local blood becomes more acidic
   - Decreased local muscle tone (skeletal & visceral)
   - Connective tissue becomes less dense & more fluid-like
   - Wound healing is accelerated

2. Systemic
   - Decreased systemic blood pressure
   - Increased heart rate and stroke volume
   - Blood volume shift from deep tissues to superficial circulation
   - Increased oxygen content of blood
   - Diaphoresis occurs with fluid & electrolyte loss

3. Reflex
   - Increased cutaneous circulation in associated reflex area
   - Increased deep tissue circulation in associated reflex area
   - Consensual or remote heating in associated reflex area
   - (see local effects of heat -- above)
   - Reflex effects may be segmental (dermatomal) in nature or be associated with somato-visceral or viscero-somatic pathways.

Effects
of Cold:

1. Local: (effects are longer lasting & deeper due to vasoconstriction)
   Decreased cellular metabolic rate
   Vasoconstriction
   Decreased vascular permeability
   Decreased blood flow to area
   Blanching of skin with piloerection
   Decreased diapedesis
   Increased leukocytosis
   Increased chemotaxis
   Increased phagocytosis
   Local blood becomes more alkaline
   Increased local muscle tone (skeletal & visceral)
   Connective tissue becomes more dense or gel-like
   Decreased neuronal activity
   Analgesia
   Wound healing is slowed

2. Systemic
   Increased systemic blood pressure initially -- progressing to
   decreased systemic blood pressure with continued cooling
   Decreased heart rate and stroke volume
   Blood volume shift from superficial to deep tissues
   Decreased oxygen content of blood
   Hypothermia

3. Reflex
   Decreased cutaneous circulation in associated reflex area
   Decreased deep tissue circulation in associated reflex area
   Consensual or remote cooling in associated reflex area
   (see local effects of cold -- above)
   Reflex effects may be segmental (dermatomal) in nature or be
   associated with somato-visceral or viscero-somatic pathways.

* Reflex responses to an application of cold also include an adaptive
heating reaction with vasodilation (aka: hunting response), which
represents an attempt by the organism to maintain homeostasis.

Effects of Contrast:

Local effects of contrast heat and cold treatments are stimulating
and increase local circulation.
Systemic effects of contrast heat and cold treatments are
stimulating and increase systemic circulation.
Reflex effects of contrast heat and cold treatments mirror the
applications of both heat and cold, yet with amplified results due to
the greater differences between applications & tissue temperature.

VIII. THERAPEUTIC TECHNIQUES AND PROCEDURES

A. Introduction

Deciding which thermal modality to use demands knowledge of the effects of either hot or cold on the involved tissue. Which modality can improve the condition of the tissue or systems? Some conditions respond better to superficial heat, and others to deep heat or cold. For example, the limited range of motion of a joint may be caused by several conditions - edema, soft-tissue contractures, muscle tension, pain/spasms, peripheral nerve damage and spasticity, or other conditions affecting the central nervous system. It is important to understand the condition and know what effect either heat or cold will have on the joint, its structure, and associated skin and musculature.

The following treatments are not all inclusive. A thorough understanding of the principles of hydrotherapy, the effects of heat and cold on the body, and the patient's health and medical conditions is necessary before attempting to use any of these treatments. Caution should be exercised. When working with the very young, elderly, or anyone with debilitative conditions or anyone currently under a physician's care, always consult with his/her physician before using these techniques.

Remember: before beginning always explain the treatment and procedures to the patient. Allow the patient time to rest and recover after the treatment. Make sure they do not chill and that any hot applications are not extreme. The patient's comfort is extremely important. Carefully document your treatment and the results.

B. Local Applications

Local applications are those, which are used over a specific body area. They are generally used to draw blood to an area (derivation), to push blood out of an area (revulsion), to stimulate the skin or body part, or to produce a numbing effect.

Cold Compress

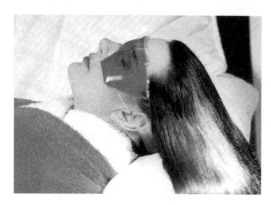

Courtesy of Corso Enterprises Inc.

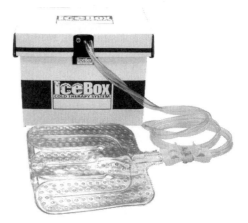

Courtesy of Orthocare

- **Description:** A treatment as simple as using a cloth wrung from cold or ice water applied to any part of the body surface. May also involve the use of chemical packs cooled in a freezer (above left) or very sophisticated self-refrigerating packs, which are designed to be form fitting for each part of the body (above right).

- **Rationale:** To decrease blood flow locally, distally, and decrease local metabolism by vasoconstriction and local hypothermia.

- **Equipment:** A wash cloth or hand towel, tailoring the size to the body part being treated, container of cold or ice water, plastic or rubber sheeting for bed or pillow. Chemical packs, self-cooling packs.

- **Procedure:** Make sure the patient is in a comfortable position; do not cover cold compress; be aware of the reflex effects of a cold application and patient sensitivity to cold. Apply the compress and press firmly. * Note the directions for use with chemical and self-cooling packs - some are not designed to directly contact the skin. Typical treatment is 20 to 30 minutes, check patient for prolonged ischemia & "hunting response," repeat as needed. Do not chill the patient. Dry the patient thoroughly after the treatment.

- **Indications:** Relieve congestion (edema), heat, redness, and pain associated with acute trauma, or following surgery and to reduce fever if applied over 1/4 of the body surface or over major vessels.

- **Contraindications:** Cold sensitivity, chilled patient, or someone who cannot give you feedback about the treatment.

Sinus Pack

- **Description:** A small cold pack is placed across the nose, lying on the face and cheeks.

- **Rationale:** To constrict the engorged blood vessels of the sinus area, causing a revulsion of blood from the area to reduce sinus congestion and pain.

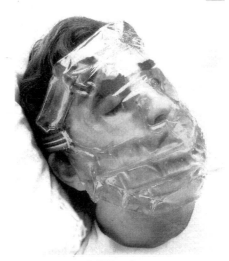

Full Face Compress -
Courtesy of Corso Enterprises Inc.

- **Equipment:** Facial compress, 2 ice packs or small towels filled with ice cubes; fomentations; cold packs; hot foot bath; towels; ice water.

- **Procedure:** Have the patient recline and place his or her feet into the hot foot bath. Perform 3 sets of contrast applications to the chest - hot fomentations for 3 minutes and cold packs for 30 seconds. Place a hot fomentation on the chest for the remainder of the treatment. Place one ice pack on the back of the neck and one on top of the head. Fold and place a small towel over the face leaving the tip of the nose exposed. Apply a small fomentation over the face towel for approximately 3 minutes. Remove the fomentation and towel. Dip another small towel in ice water and drape it over the face in the same way. Leave on for 30 seconds. Repeat the face fomentation - cold compress sequence 3 times. Remove the cold compress and dry the face.

- **Indications:** Congestive headache, upper respiratory infection.

- **Contraindications:** Low blood pressure, peripheral vascular disease, and cold sensitivity.

80

Ice Pack

- **Description:** The local application of cold over a covered body part. There are many uses for ice packs, all based on the same principles.

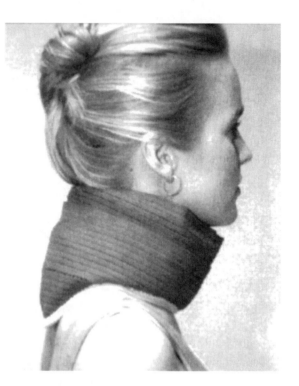

- **Rationale:** Applications of prolonged cold initially constrict, then dilate and finally constrict the area. Circulation is decreased (by retrostasis). Swelling and congestion are reduced. The metabolic process is slowed down and pain is reduced.

- **Equipment:** Towel, ice bag filled with crushed ice, or a ready-made cold pack. There are a number of ready-made cold packs available in various sizes and shapes for convenience, or you can use a "homemade" pack.

- **Procedure:** Cover the body part with a towel. Place the ice pack over the towel for 20 - 30 minutes at a time, check patient for prolonged ischemia & "hunting response," repeat as needed. Remove the ice pack and towel. Dry the area.

- **Indications:** Acute sprains, strains; acute joint inflammation; acute bursitis; headaches; backache; tennis elbow; areas of inflammation and swelling; acute appendicitis; over the heart if the beat is rapid (tachycardia); fever; sinus congestion.

- **Contraindications:** Adverse reactions to cold; over lungs if the patient has acute asthma; over the heart with bradycardia, and an extremely chilly patient.

Cold Foot Bath

- **Description:** A cold foot bath requires briefly soaking the feet and ankles in cold to very cold water.

- **Rationale:** Used for any condition requiring a reflex contraction of blood vessels of the pelvic organs, bladder, gastrointestinal tract, liver, or brain. It also helps to control post-partum bleeding, or bleeding from the kidney or bladder.

- **Equipment:** One bath or foot tub with water between 40 and 60 degrees F; towel.

- **Procedure:** Pour cold water into foot tub up to 4 inches in depth. Ask the patient to place his or her feet into the tub for 20 seconds to 2 minutes. The feet may be massaged or the patient may walk in place during the treatment if desired. Have the patient remove their feet from the tub and dry thoroughly. Allow to patient to rest.

- **Indications:** To stimulate abdominal and pelvic organs and control post-partum bleeding, or kidney or bladder bleeding.

- **Contraindications:** Asthma; acute pulmonary inflammations; chilled patient; during a headache (particularly vascular headache).

Ice Massage

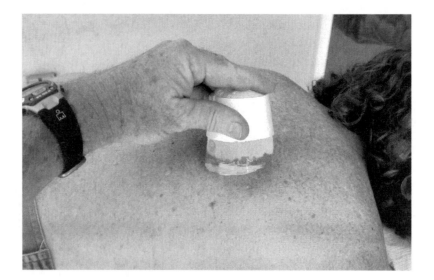

- **Description:** Ice massage is the application of ice with deep circular friction over a small area (best if trigger point is present).

- **Rationale:** An application of prolonged cold initially causes vasoconstriction, then vasodilation. Circulation initially decreases and then it will increase. Swelling and congestion are reduced. Pain is decreased via the "gate theory" (hyperstimulation analgesia) from cold, friction and pressure, and the pain-spasm-ischemia cycle is broken.

- **Equipment:** Ice; cloth. A foam cup with water frozen inside is an excellent tool for ice massage. Simply peel the cup back as the ice melts.

- **Procedure:** Apply ice over the small area being treated with deep circular massage. Keep the massage continuous and smooth for approximately 5 to 15 minutes. The patient will first feel cold, followed by slight burning, then deeper aching, and finally numbness. Treatment is complete when the area is numb and blood has rushed in. Pat dry area softly with the cloth.

- **Indications:** Acute pain; active trigger points which refer pain; muscle spasm; decreased muscle tone; inflammation and swelling.

- **Contraindications:** Adverse reaction to cold; skin sensitivity.

Contrast to Head

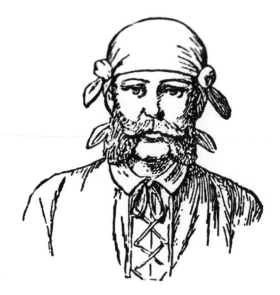

- **Description:** Alternating heat and cold applications are applied to the head. The application of heat is a key ingredient in this treatment because it produces a derivative effect.

- **Rationale:** Improve cerebral circulation by vascular stimulation. Cold initiates vasoconstriction while heat initiates vasodilation.

- **Equipment:** Covered oblong ice pack or two small ice packs, ice, two compresses (towels may be used), two sets of fomentations (a room treatment will require 6 fomentations to make 3 changes), material for hot foot bath, plastic sheet, towels, basin of ice water, shower cap, drape sheet or blanket, hospital-type gown.

- **Procedure:** Cover bed and pillow with plastic sheet. Begin with hot foot bath beginning at 105 degrees F and increase as needed (not to exceed 105 degrees F). Place a fomentation (or hot water bottle) covered with a towel under cervical spine and side of neck; place a compress wrung from ice water on the face, covering the top of the head and ears. Press down firmly over the forehead and temporal arteries, *renewing every minute*; replace the fomentation to the neck with an ice pack or two covered ice bags; replace cold compress to the face with a fomentation or towel wrung from hot water; cover ears and forehead leaving nose area open, allowing the patient to breathe fresh air; protect the eyes from excessive heat. Repeat these procedures 3 times. In other words:

| Step 1..... | Fomentation to Neck | Cold compress to Face | 3 minutes |
| | Ice to Neck | Fomentation to Face | 3 minutes |

| Step 2..... | Fomentation to Neck | Cold Compress to Face | 3 minutes |
| | Ice to Neck | Fomentation to Face | 3 minutes |

| Step 3..... | Fomentation to Neck | Cold Compress to Face | 3 minutes |
| | Ice to Neck | Fomentation to Face | 3 minutes |

Do not press down on the fomentation; continue to alternate treatments - completing three sets of heat and cold; hold the feet above a foot tub, pour cold water over feet and then dry; cool face by sponging with a cold compress, dry patient thoroughly after treatment, especially hair. Allow patient to rest at least 30 minutes after treatment and avoid chilling. Record treatment and reactions.

- Indications: Headaches due to congestion of common cold, nervous and muscular tension, and certain headaches associated with trauma or muscle tension.

- Contraindications: History of migraine or other vascular headaches. History of aneurysm or glaucoma. Use precaution on patients with a history of cardiovascular disease or inner ear disorders.

Contrast to Chest

- **Description:** Alternate heat and cold applications are applied to the chest. If heat is applied to the lower extremities, systemic derivation will also occur.

- **Rationale:** Vascular stimulation.

- **Equipment:** 5 towels, 2 compress cloths, 2 small rubber sheets, bath blanket, large piece of ice and bath basin, and 5 fomentations in container well wrapped to minimize heat loss.

- **Procedures:** Explain procedure, assemble materials, protect bed and drape patient with bath blanket. Help patient turn on his/her side. Place rubber sheet, one fomentation and bath towel lengthwise as close as possible beside patient's back. Have patient turn back on the fomentation, making sure that the fomentation is smooth and not too hot; cover the chest with a towel and place a fomentation over the towel. Cover patient with a bath blanket and place a rubber sheet, a fomentation and a towel under the patient's feet. Wrap well, covering them with a bath blanket. Remove the fomentation from the chest and have the patient breath deeply while the chest is rubbed briskly with ice (repeat two times). Dry area thoroughly and apply the next fomentation. Make three applications of heat and cold to the chest, finishing with cold. Remove the fomentations from the feet and back and cool the parts with alcohol and dry thoroughly. The entire treatment should take only l0 to l5 minutes. Make sure the patient is thoroughly dry upon completion of the treatment. Make a record of the treatment and results.

- **Indications:** Stimulate respiration and recovery from anesthesia and prevent circulatory stasis, chest cold, and chest congestion in some surgical cases.

- **Contraindications:** Not recommended for children under l2 years of age, special care with older patients, as well as diabetics.

Eye Compress

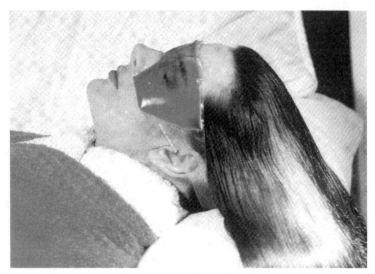

Courtesy of Corso Enterprises Inc

- Description: A hot or cold compress is applied to the eyes.

- Rationale: Cold decreases blood flow to area, and heat increases blood flow, as well as the metabolism.

- Equipment: Cotton, bowl, gauze or small cloth, wooden spoon.

- Procedures: Place cotton on end of wooden spoon and wrap a piece of gauze or small cloth around the cotton and tie in place. Dip the cotton into hot or cold water, pressing out the excess water. Place the compress over the eye. Hold in place for up to 20 minutes. It may be necessary to repeat every 3 to 4 hours.

- Indications: Acute glaucoma and iridocycitis, sty, and minor infections.

- Contraindications: Cold or heat sensitivity, cancer, diabetic retinopathy.

Hot Compress (Hot Pack)

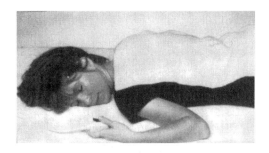

- Description: A moist hot compress or hot pack is also known as a **fomentation** and includes the local application of moist heat to a body surface using a blanket like cloth. The cloth is usually 50% cotton and 50% wool to retain water. An electric moist heating pad, known as a thermophore*, may also be used.

- Rationale: To increase blood flow to local tissues, promote leukocytosis, diapadesis and chemotaxis, promote diaphoresis, relax superficial musculature and white connective tissue, and produce tissue warming prior to another modality such as massage.

- Equipment: Cotton / wool cloths; towel(s); water heated to desired temperature. *Thermophore; towel(s).

- Procedure: Cover the area being treated with several layers of towels. Place the heated cloth over the towels. Cover hot pack with several layers of dry towel or blanket. Remove compress after a period of 20 - 30 minutes. Do not allow patient to lie on the hot pack. Always be certain that the patient is comfortable and the fomentation is not too hot. Remove the compress, dry the area, and have the patient rest or repeat the treatment as necessary.

- Indications: Muscle spasms, tension and soreness; areas of decreased blood flow; decreased range of motion; relieve joint pain and inflammation in rheumatic fever, chronic arthritis, or synovitis; Reduce congestion from chest cold, pharyngitis, laryngitis, tonsillitis, chronic bronchitis, whooping cough, or pneumonia; reduce pain from stomach disorders, prostatitis, cystitis, dysmenorrhea (menstrual cramps), renal colic, or sciatica (to name a few); help reduce nervous tension and insomnia; prior to massage or other modalities.

- Contraindications: Over areas of acute inflammation (acute injuries) or bleeding; patients w/ congestive heart failure; peripheral vascular disease, loss of sensation; malignant (cancerous) tumors; or gastric ulcers.

Hot Foot Bath

- **Description:** A hot foot bath requires soaking the feet and ankles in water ranging from 100 to 110 degrees F. It is one of the simplest and most frequently employed techniques. It is often used as part of a treatment such as the Russian bath.

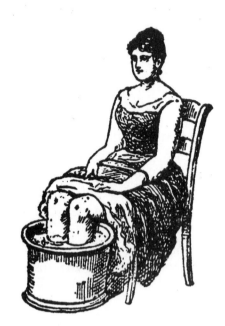

- **Rationale:** Causes local and reflex increases in blood flow through the feet and entire skin surface, producing decongestion in internal organs and brain.

- **Equipment:** Chair; blanket or towel; foot tub and a cold compress.

- **Procedure:** Have the patient relax comfortably in the chair. Fill the foot tub with water at the desired temperature. Touch the water with your hand to test the temperature before allowing the patient to place their feet into the tub. Have the patient place his or her feet into the water; making sure the water covers their ankles too. Drape the blanket or towel over the patient's lap, and over the foot tub. Treatment time is between 10 and 30 minutes. Add more hot water as necessary to maintain the temperature. Apply the cold compress to the patient's forehead or to the back of the neck so their head does not become congested or over-heated. When the treatment is complete, have the patient remove their feet from the foot bath and momentarily rinse their feet with cool water. Pat dry. Allow patient to rest.

- **Indications:** Congestive headache; relieve pelvic congestion; nosebleeds (epistaxis); relieve congestion of internal organs such as the lungs; produce a general warming of the body to get rid of a chill; help prevent or relieve the common cold; help reduce plantar warts.

- **Contraindications:** Loss of sensation, diabetes, peripheral vascular disease - arteriosclerosis.

Contrast Foot Bath

- **Description:** A contrast foot or local bath requires alternately soaking the feet and ankles in a series of hot (100°-110°F) and cold (40°-70°F) baths. This is a powerful therapy, yet simple in its application.

- **Rationale:** This treatment may be used for any condition requiring an increase in circulation, or in conditions where the internal organs are congested and blood needs to be shunted to the lower extremities. The application of heat causes vasodilation, while short cold applications lead to an immediate vasoconstriction, followed by reflexive vasodilation. The overall effect is one of creating a pumping action.

- **Equipment:** Two tubs or tanks of appropriate size; hot and cold water; a bath thermometer; towels; and disinfectant.

- **Procedure:** Fill the first tub with hot water (103°F) and antiseptic (if open wounds are present). Place body parts in hot bath for 3 minutes. Fill the second tub with cold water. Place body parts in cold bath for 30 seconds. Repeat step one, but increase hot water temperature by 2 degrees to 105°F. Repeat cold procedure for 30 seconds. Repeat previous steps increasing each hot application by 1-2 degrees until a water temp of 110 ° is reached. Each hot application should be 3 minutes in length and followed by 30 seconds of cold. Use at least 3 hot/cold cycles, but no more than 6, as the intensity of the reaction decreases beyond that point. Dry thoroughly and have the patient rest for 30 minutes.

- **Indications:** Local infections, non-acute and chronic traumatic injuries, bruises, arthritis, edema, venous stasis, and ulcers.

- **Contraindications:** Cancer, peripheral vascular disease (Diabetes), diminished sensation or inability to report, and hemorrhage.

Hydrocollator (Chemical Pack)

- **Description:** A hydrocollator is a small metal tank used to heat water to 150 - 160 degrees F. Chemical packs of silica gel are placed into the tank of heated water. When the pack reaches the desired temperature, it is ready for use as a local application of moist heat.

- **Rationale:** Increase blood flow to local tissues, promote leukocytosis, diapedesis and chemotaxis, promote diaphoresis, relax superficial musculature and white connective tissue, and provide tissue warming prior to another modality such as massage.

- **Equipment:** Hydrocollator tank containing water heated to 150 - 160 degrees F; silica gel pack(s); several towels or terry cloth covers.

- **Procedure:** Place six layers of towel over area to be treated. Carefully remove a heated gel pack from the hydrocollator and place on top of the towel. Cover the outer surface with several layers of towels. If using terry cloth covers, insert pack into cover, apply to area, and cover with towel. Leave on the area for 20 - 30 minutes. Do not allow patient to lie on pack. Take care that the patient does not get over-heated and starts perspiring. Remove the pack and towels. Dry the area. Allow patient to rest.

- **Indications:** Muscle spasm and related pain, decreased range of motion.

- **Contraindications:** Over areas of acute inflammation or bleeding; myocardial infarction (heart attack); loss of sensation (from diabetes or paralysis); malignant tumors; gastric ulcers.

Paraffin Bath

- **Description:** A paraffin bath is a local application of melted paraffin wax to the skin surface. The paraffin delivers heat very effectively to painful joints or body parts and leaves the skin smooth, soft, and pliable.

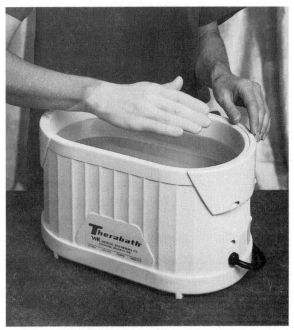

Paraffin Bath - Courtesy of Therabath

- **Rationale:** To produce hyperemia as well as increase blood flow to local tissues; promote leukocytosis, diapedesis and chemotaxis; to promote diaphoresis; relax superficial musculature and white connective tissue; and produce tissue warming.

- **Equipment:** Heating unit; 5 lbs paraffin wax; 1 pint mineral oil; thermometer.

- **Procedure:** Melt the paraffin and mineral oil in the double boiler. Bring the temperature of the mixture to 122 - 130 degrees F. Examine the body part to be treated to make sure there are no lesions or open wounds. Wash and dry the body part. Instruct the patient to dip the body part into the mixture, holding the area relaxed to avoid cracks in the paraffin. Allow a few seconds of cooling time between each application. If the area cannot be dipped, take some paraffin and "paint" it over the body part. Leave the paraffin on for 20 - 30 minutes. A plastic bag or towel may be wrapped around it to conserve heat. Remove the paraffin and discard.

- **Indications:** For use over arthritic or stiff joints (possibly after a fracture or a sprain has occurred, but not in its acute phase); bursitis; fibrositis; gout; preparation for massage.

- **Contraindications:** Acute injury, local infection, diabetes w/PVD, cancer.

C. Rubs and Inhalations

Steam Inhalation

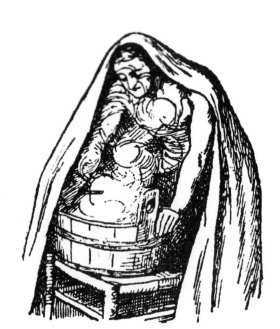

- Description: Steam inhalation provides a moist, hot treatment for the lungs and entire respiratory tract. Even though commercial vaporizers are readily available, a "makeshift" treatment will provide the same benefits.

- Rationale: Heating the mucosa increases circulation to the respiratory tract and decreases congestion. Expectoration is increased. Aromatic oils, if used, increase penetration and add their own medicinal effects, as well as the psychological benefits of the fragrances.

- Equipment: Vaporizer (or tea kettle or pot with boiling water); sheet or towel; aromatic oils, if desired; umbrella; cool damp cloth.

- Procedure: Heat vaporizer or bring water in the kettle or pot to a boil. Add aromatic oils if desired. Position the patient over the rising steam, making sure that it is not too hot. Open the umbrella and position over the patient's head. Place a towel or sheet over the umbrella, making a tent over the patient and the steam. Advise the patient to breathe slowly and deeply. Wipe the patient's face with a cool damp cloth as needed. The patient may continue to breathe the moist steam for 30 - 60 minutes up to three times a day. When treatment is completed, dry the patient and let him or her rest.

- Indications: Congestion of the respiratory tract; cough; sore throat; laryngitis; heavy mucous.

- Contraindications: Congestive heart failure; any serious heart problems; heat sensitivity.

Alcohol Rub

- Description: The application of rubbing alcohol to the surface of the body with friction.

- Rationale: Friction brings blood to the superficial tissues and as the alcohol evaporates, heat is liberated from the body. Note: without friction, the skin would become chilled and blood would move to deeper tissue preventing any appreciable heat loss.

- Equipment: Rubbing alcohol 70% solution; (water if using 90% alcohol).

- Procedure: Pour alcohol into cupped hands (Dilute a solution of alcohol using 2/3 alcohol to 1/3 water - if using 90% alcohol). Begin with the arm, rubbing with upward strokes. Use short alternating strokes for a cooling effect and to aid in the evaporation of the alcohol. After treating the upper extremities, apply to chest, lower extremities and back.

- Indications: Fever reduction; for a cooling effect after applications of heat; refresh patient if a bath is not given.

- Contraindications: Chilled patient, open lesions, extremely weak patient.

94

D. Full Body Packs

Hot Blanket Pack

- **Description:**
This is a full body wrap of blankets and fomentations to produce mild hyperthermia and profuse sweating.

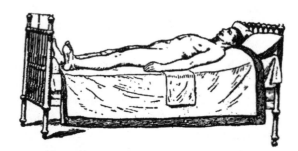

- **Rationale:**
To elevate the body temperature to produce a mild to moderate fever. As circulation increases there is a great influx of white blood cells in the bloodstream. This procedure stimulates the production of antibodies, increases diapadesis, chemotaxis, and phagocytosis; thus increasing the immune response to fight infection.

- **Equipment:**
Four blankets; 2 plastic sheets; 1 sheet; towels; fomentation packs or an electric blanket; cold compress.

- **Procedure:**
Place three blankets on a bed and cover with a plastic sheet. Lay several fomentation packs on the sheet, enough to extend from the patient's neck to the thighs. An electric blanket may be used instead of fomentation packs. Wrap the patient in a sheet. Let them lie on the fomentation packs, securing them along both sides. Place another fomentation pack over the abdomen and one on the feet. Place another plastic sheet over the patient and a blanket on top. Place a cold compress on the forehead. Allow the patient to rest from 45 minutes to several hours. Take the patient's temperature and pulse every 15 minutes and make sure that the skin is not overheating. If the pulse nears 160 beats per minute or the temperature goes over 104 degrees F, stop the treatment. Sweating will be very heavy. Give the patient fluids as necessary. Remove the patient from the packs. Have he or she take a shower or administer a sponge bath.

- **Indications:**
Systemic infection, Cold, Flu, Rheumatoid arthritis, Colic, any condition in which sweating and vasodilation are desirable.

© Pine Island Publishers Inc. 2003

- Contraindications: Congestive heart failure; history of heat stroke; advanced age, claustrophobia, diabetes, peripheral vascular disease, grave illness, severe anemia, or an extremely weak patient.

Wet Sheet Pack

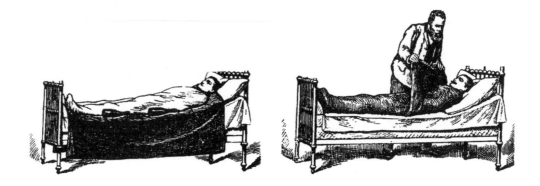

- Description: This is a full-body wrap with a cold, wet sheet wrapped directly around the patient with several layers of dry blankets on the outside. The dry blankets are placed on top of the patient to help regulate the temperature of the treatment and the amount of evaporation required.

- Rationale: Used to increase metabolism and circulation and to encourage hyperthermia and sweating. The cold application to the skin stimulates a heating response ("hunting response"), which continues as the water evaporates. The greater the area of skin stimulated by cold, the greater the heating reaction. As the patient responds to the treatment, varied reactions occur including: stimulation, sedation, hyperthermia, and lastly, diaphoresis.

- Equipment: One sheet; 2 wool blankets; hot packs; cold compress; towels; pillow.

- Procedure: Soak sheet in cold water and wring out. Wrap the patient in the sheet and let them lie down on his back, head resting on a pillow. Wrap the dry wool blanket on top of the wet sheet and tuck in around patient, using additional blankets as needed. Apply hot packs to the feet to be sure that the patient stays warm. Apply a cold compress to the head as necessary and offer water to drink. When the treatment is complete, unwrap the patient and apply cold mitten friction. Allow the patient to rest in dry bedding for 30 minutes. The duration of treatment may vary from 30 minutes to eight hours, depending on the desired response.

- Indications: 1st stage: fever; weakness, anemia, general debilitated states.
                  2nd stage: depression, mania, insomnia, nervousness, indigestion.
                  3rd stage: constipation, nephritis, liver congestion, irritable bowel, ulcerative colitis, Crohn's disease, malabsorption, and pneumonia.
                  4th stage: cold, flu, bronchitis, addictions, Liver disease, measles, and as a preventive measure.

- Contraindications: Diabetes; very severe colds or flu; skin conditions made worse by moisture; acute asthma; claustrophobia; cardiovascular disease; extreme weakness; chilled patient;
                  * Use caution with very young or very old patient.

Speisman Pack (Modified Wet Sheet Pack)

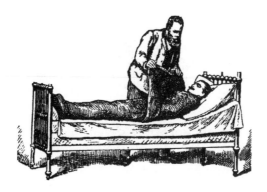

- **Description:** Dr. Speisman modified the wet sheet pack to specifically treat cases of pneumonia.

- **Rationale:** To encourage hyperthermia and increase the general immune response (as in the before mentioned treatment), specifically to increase the quantity and quality of blood flow to and from the lower respiratory tract.

- **Equipment:** One sheet; 1 box Epsom Salts; 1 wool blanket; 1 electric blanket; 1 dry towel.

- **Procedure:** Soak sheet in cold water with Epsom Salt solution and wring out. Wrap the patient in the wet sheet, then the dry wool blanket, and finally the electric blanket. Allow him to lay down on his back comfortably. Set electric blanket at a low setting, adjusting to the vitality of the patient. Allow patient to rest quietly for 30 - 45 minutes. Monitor the temperature and pulse of the patient. Apply treatment as desired first thing in the morning. Repeat treatment as trunk pack in the afternoon and before bed. Use heated compress to the chest every other hour between Speisman packs.

- **Indications:** Lower respiratory tract infections; pneumonia; colds; flu; irritable bowel; colitis; constipation; nephritis; insomnia; hepatitis; to detoxify.

- **Contraindications:** Severe anemia; extreme weakness; diabetes; peripheral vascular disease; heart disease; claustrophobia; acute asthma.

Wet Sheet Pack - Heated

- **Description:** This is a cold wet sheet wrap applied to the trunk and hips of the body. It is considered to be one of the most important of Vincent Priessnitz's contributions.

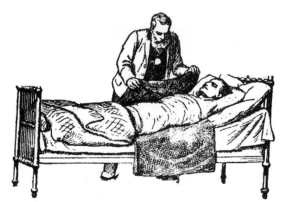

- **Rationale:** To stimulate the organs of the gastrointestinal tract and to alleviate congestive disorders of the digestive system. There are several stages; the first is cooling (5-20 minutes), second is neutral (30 to one hour), third is heating (30 minutes to one hour), and lastly is sweating (one to two hours or more). The cold stage results in constriction and dilation, increased tissue temperature, and circulation, increased derivation and congestion, increased metabolism, and increased elimination. This procedure has a tonic effect.

- **Equipment:** One sheet; 1 blanket; cold water; heated compress.

- **Procedure:** Place a blanket across a bed, wide enough to cover from the patient's neck down to their hips. Soak a sheet in cold water and wring it out. Place the wet sheet on top of the blanket. Ask the patient to lie on his back on the wet sheet. Pull one side of the sheet under the arm, across the abdomen, and secure it under the other arm. Place a hot water bottle, heating pad, or fomentation pack over the abdomen. Pull the other side of the wet sheet under the arm, across the abdomen and secure it under the other arm. Place the blanket snugly around the patient. Allow the patient to rest there for 20 - 25 minutes.

- **Indications:** Fever; indigestion; digestive disturbances; chronic liver congestion; dyspepsia; reduced gastric motility; flatulence; nausea; vomiting; some psychiatric disorders, where reduction in anxiety is the desired result.

- **Contraindications:** Anemia (heating and sweating stages), chilled patient, extremely debilitated person, acute asthma, claustrophobia, skin conditions worsened by moisture, weak heart, severe colds and flu, diabetes, or other circulatory problems.

E. Frictions

Cold Mitten Friction

- **Description:** A friction massage using mitts, cloths, towels, or a loofah sponge which has been dipped in cold water.

- **Rationale:** To increase circulation when needed to promote the elimination of heat, resulting in a decrease in internal congestion. Increased circulation brings in more red and white blood cells, which aid in the elimination of inflammatory products and increases the patient's resistance to infections. It restores normal tone to tissues and muscles, and raises energy and endurance levels.

- **Equipment:** Towels; mitts or washcloths; bowl of cold water 50 to 75 degrees F

- **Procedure:** Have the patient lie on a blanket or towel, placing a dry towel under the area to be treated. Dip the mitt or washcloth in the cold water and ring it out. Start a back and forth rubbing motion at the fingertips, working up the arm to the shoulder and back down to the fingers until the skin becomes pink. Dip the mitt into the cold water as necessary. Dry the arm with friction movements using a towel. Repeat this procedure on the other arm, chest, abdomen, and legs. Keep the areas not being treated covered and warm at all times. Ask the patient to turn over and repeat the treatment on the back, hips and legs. Make sure the patient is dry and covered. Allow him or her to rest for 30 minutes.

- **Indications:** Poor circulation; anemia; poor resistance to infections; low thyroid activity; alcoholism; fever; cold and flu prevention; low energy and endurance; depression; drug or tobacco withdrawal; finish for hot treatments.

- Contraindications: Skin infections and lesions; chilled patient; patient who cannot endure friction massage.

Salt Glow

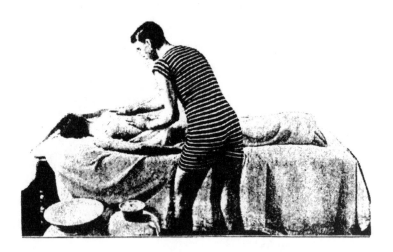

- Description: The application of moist salt with friction massage to the patient's skin. It is a labor-intensive treatment.

- Rationale: The friction results in vasodilation and increased circulation with no increase in temperature. The mechanical effects cause chemical irritations, which increase nerve and sebaceous activity and removal of superficial skin. The salt solution may cause osmosis of fluid toward the superficial tissues softening skin. It has a very tonic effect and does not rely on hot or cold. To intensify the effect in **strong** patients, the salt may be softened in ice water.

- Equipment: One to two pounds of Epsom salts (common table salt or one with a coarser grind will do); water; basin or container, towel; (chair; if necessary). *Use a hot footbath if desired (with chilled patient).

- Procedure: Moisten the salt enough to make the salt grains stick together, but not dissolve. Wet the patient's skin with water. Take both hands full of moistened salt and apply to an extremity, beginning a friction massage to the patient's tolerance. Apply treatment to the arms and legs first, starting with the fingers and toes respectively. After the extremities, apply the salt rub to the chest, abdomen, back, hips, and buttocks. Wash all of the salt off and dry patient thoroughly and briskly with a towel. * Have patient sit or lie with feet in hot bath if desired.

- Indications: To stimulate and soften and the skin and muscles; stimulate nervous system for increased vigor; chronic illnesses;

sluggish circulation; low resistance to infections. As a general
tonic - especially when patient cannot tolerate cold sheet wrap.

- Contraindications: Open skin lesions; skin irritation; same as for the hot footbath.

F. Baths

Brand Bath

- Description: A cool (to cold) immersion bath with friction to the whole body except the abdomen.

- Rationale: To dissipate heat from internal organs to the skin surface for elimination. The friction draws blood to the body surface where heat can be transferred to the water. To reduce severe fever - body temperature may decrease as much as 3 to 4 degrees F with each treatment.

- Equipment: Bath tub containing water at 70 - 80 degrees F; sponge; towels.

- Procedure: Assist the patient into the tub of cool water. Use a sponge to the body surface and rub vigorously for 2 to 3 minutes. Have the patient sit up and pour cool water over the head. Have the patient lie back and rub vigorously for another 5 minutes. Continue the rub and cool water pouring for 10 to 30 minutes (or until fever is reduced). Cease treatment if patient begins to shiver (as this will cause temperature to rise). Assist the patient out of the tub, dry, wrap in a blanket and allow to rest. * Hydrate patient.

- Indications: High fever (105 degrees F or above) when lassitude, restlessness, delirium, or shallow breathing are present. This is a heroic treatment and should be used only when more conservative treatments (Dry friction, Warm bath, Tepid bath or shower with friction, Hot sheet Pack) have failed.

- Contraindications: Chilled patient who is shivering or patient with mild fever.

Cold Short Bath

- **Description:** A bath with cold water and friction.

- **Rationale:** Cold and friction are both stimulating eliciting a generalized nervous and circulatory system response. To help reduce fever and as a general immune stimulant. A general tonic treatment

- **Equipment:** Tub with water from 55 - 90 degrees F.; towel; coarse washcloth.

- **Procedure:** Assist the patient into the tub. Begin massaging (friction) at once with a coarse washcloth. Treatment time may be from 30 seconds at colder temperatures to 20 minutes at warmer temperatures. Constantly massage the skin to keep the blood flowing actively. Assist the patient from the tub and dry briskly with a dry towel.

- **Indications:** High fevers (as in the cases of malaria and typhoid); multiple sclerosis; colds; flu; rheumatic fever; lupus erythematous. Used daily as a tonic in patients with slow metabolism.

- **Contraindications:** Chilled patient, very weak patient.

Hubbard Tank

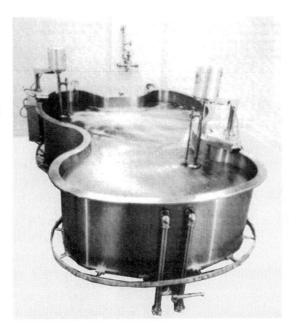

- Description: A specially constructed full-immersion tub with a turbine for administering underwater exercises with neutral or mild heat.

- Rationale: To produce a mild increase in circulation when needed to aid in mobilization of joints. It is relaxing and does not put too much stress on the patient. This treatment will aid in stretching and exercise as well as provide a cleansing effect for the treatment of burns or decubitus ulcers.

- Equipment: Hubbard tank with water between 90 and 100 degrees F.; towels.

- Procedure: Assist the patient into the tank. Direct the turbine at the specific areas for hydromassage. After several minutes of using the turbine and the treatment area is sufficiently warmed, assist the patient with stretching and range of motion exercises. The treatment time is 20 - 30 minutes. Assist the patient from the tank and dry thoroughly. Allow them to rest.

- Indications: Rheumatoid arthritis; neuromuscular conditions, such as hemiplegia, poliomyelitis, Parkinson's disease, multiple sclerosis, and cerebral palsy; postoperative orthopedic conditions; burns; and decubitus ulcers.

- Contraindications: Respiratory or cardiovascular insufficiency.

Medicated Bath

- **Description:** There are a number of substances, which may be added to a neutral temperature bath to enhance specific therapeutic effects. These include: Aveeno (oatmeal), cornstarch, and baking soda.

- **Rationale:** The soothing properties of these substances, combined with the non-stimulating neutral temperature of the water, tend to decrease the amount and intensity of nerve impulses originating from the skin.

- **Equipment:** Two cups Aveeno or finely ground oatmeal, or two cups dry corn starch, or one pound baking soda (sodium bicarbonate).

- **Procedure:** Mix any of the above with 30 gallons of neutral water. Allow the patient to sit in the solution from 10-30 minutes. Finish bath by patting patient dry (do not rub with towel).
  Caution - Aveeno makes bottom of tub slippery.

- **Indications:** Skin irritations from insect bites, contact dermatitis, sunburn, hives, chafing and eczema.

- **Contraindications:** Open wounds and contagious skin conditions.

*Other herbal and pharmaceutical substances available as bath additives are listed in the following chart:

Substance	Effect
Apple Cider Vinegar	Restores natural Ph to skin
Bran	Softens the skin
Fennel & Nettle	Mild detoxifier/cleanser
Ginger	Improves circulation and diaphoretic
Hayflower	Releases skin impurities
Nutmeg	Diaphoretic/cleanser
Pine	Good for rashes and open sores, softens and stimulates skin
Rosemary	Stimulates blood circulation
Oatstraw	Releases skin impurities
Sage	Stimulates sweat glands

Mud Bath

- **Description:** A covering of the entire body in mud, clay, or other earth products containing antibacterial properties.

- **Rationale:** The antibacterial properties of mud help to discourage infection, improve blood circulation to the skin, stimulate metabolism, help to decrease inflammatory masses, and promote tissue repair.

- **Equipment:** A bath tub or cot; shower curtain or plastic sheet; mud (clay); water; towel.

- **Procedure:** Place the shower curtain or plastic sheet into a bathtub or over a cot. Mix the mud with the desired temperature of water to make a soft consistency. Place a sufficient amount of mud in the tub or on the sheet. Allow the patient to sit in the tub or on the sheet and assist them in dipping the mud on all parts of the body and face. Let them lie down and continue to cover the body with mud to about 1/2 to 2/3rds of an inch thick. Treatment time may be from 20 minutes to 4 - 6 hours. When the desired length of time is over, assist the patient up and help brush off the excess mud. The patient then takes a shower or bath and is allowed to rest.

- **Indications:** Pain; swelling; infections; arthritis; gout; eczema; poison ivy; dermatological diseases; retention of wastes in the kidney due to kidney failure; cancer; lupus.

- **Contraindications:** Open wounds and contagious skin conditions.

106

Neutral Bath

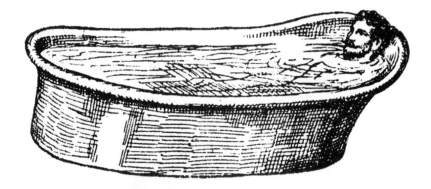

- **Description:**   Immersion of the whole body in a tub of water at neutral temperatures (94 to 98 degrees F).

- **Rationale:**   The neutral temperature felt by the body relaxes nervous impulses to and from the brain, producing a sedative, relaxed feeling. It creates an equalizing effect on the circulatory system.

- **Equipment:**   Tub of water at 94 - 98 degrees F, towels.

- **Procedure:**   Assist the patient into the tub, placing a pillow or towel under the head for comfort. Allow the patient to lie quietly and relax. They may stay there for 15 to 60 minutes, or for conditions such as insomnia, up to 3 - 4 hours. Stay with the patient for the duration of treatment. Add warm water to maintain the temperature. Assist the patient out of the tub and dry gently. Let him have undisturbed rest.

- **Indications:**   Insomnia; irritability; anxiety; depression; fever; acute high blood pressure; edema in the outer areas of the body; drug withdrawal; pregnancy toxemia; chronic pain; itching.

- **Contraindications:** Skin conditions aggravated by water such as eczema; serious cardiac weakness.

Russian Bath

- Description:

A body steam
bath given
with the head
not exposed to
the steam.
Historically,
the patient is
reclining.
There are a
number
of portable and
permanent
installations
available.

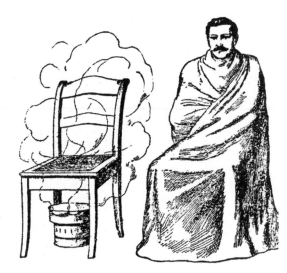

- Rationale:

Used when an increase in metabolism and circulation is needed.
The resulting dilation of blood vessels increases blood flow and
produces tissue relaxation. Also, with an increase in metabolism,
there is an increase in body temperature causing sweating and
encouraging an elimination of metabolic byproducts. There is no
heat lost in this procedure due to 100% humidity.

- Equipment:

Steam room; table; cold compress; towel or blanket. (A makeshift Russian Bath can be made with a chair, tea kettle with boiling
water, hot plate and two blankets to cover the patient up to the
neck.)

- Procedure:

Cover the patient with a blanket or towel and assist him or her into
the steam room. The temperature inside should be between 110 -
120 degrees F. Have them lay down on their back with their head
outside of the room. Place a cold compress around the neck.
Another cold compress may be placed over the heart if the heart
rate is too rapid. Allow the patient to rest comfortably for 5 to 10
minutes (they may stay in for as long as 20 minutes). Take the
patient's pulse every 5 minutes and give them cool water to drink
as necessary. If a steam room is not available, have the patient sit
in a wooden or plastic chair and place the kettle of hot water on a
hot plate under the chair, making sure that the spout is not directly
pointed at the patient. Drape the patient in one blanket from the
front, and one blanket from the neck to the floor in back.

Take all precautions not to burn the patient or allow the blankets to catch fire. Assist the patient from the steam room or chair and allow them to take a short cold shower. If a shower is not available, apply cold mitten friction and pour cold water over the feet. Cover the patient warmly and allow them to rest for at least 30 minutes.

- Indications: To produce a short, mild fever with sweating; colds and flu; rheumatoid arthritis; gout; jaundice; hypotension; insomnia; nervousness; sinus congestion or congestive headache; general relaxation, or in preparation for massage.

- Contraindications: Hypertension; diabetes; anemia; heart disease; peripheral vascular disease (i.e. arteriosclerosis); decreased sensitivity; weakness; and pregnancy.

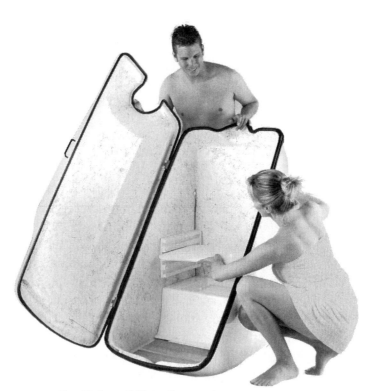

Portable Steam Cabinet - Courtesy of Steam Embrace

Steam Bath

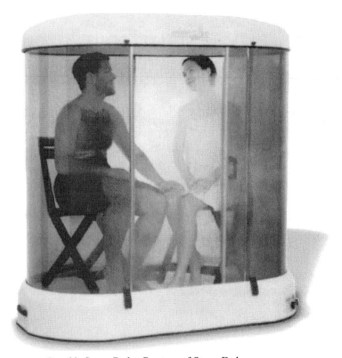

Portable Steam Bath - Courtesy of Steam Embrace

- Description: Similar to Russian bath, but with full body exposed to steam often referred to as a "steam room." Patient may be sitting or reclining. * The equipment, procedures, indications, and contraindications are similar to those for the Russian bath described above.

Sauna

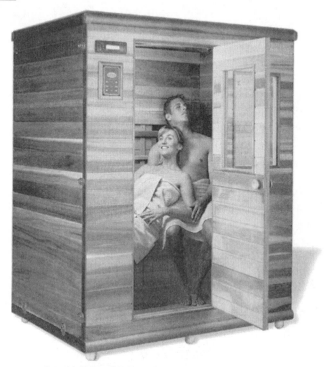

Portable Infrared Sauna - Courtesy of Steam Embrace

- Description: Full body application of heat in a dry environment. The
                     temperature is typically regulated at 180-190 degrees F (100-130
                     F for the Infrared Sauna). The lack of moisture in the air limits
                     the amount of heat transferred to the body by conduction.

- Equipment: Sauna cabinet or room. Traditional saunas are heated by wood
                     stoves and are lined with either cedar or redwood. Cold water and
                     cloth.

- Procedure: Gradually increase patient's time in sauna from 3 - 4 minutes
                     to 15-20 minutes. Apply cold water with cloth liberally to head.
                     End with cool or cold rinse.

- Indications: To produce a short, mild fever with sweating; colds and flu;
                     rheumatoid arthritis; gout; jaundice; hypotension; insomnia;
                     nervousness; sinus congestion or congestive headache; general
                     relaxation; or in preparation for massage.

- Contraindications: Hypertension; diabetes; anemia; heart disease; peripheral vascular
                     disease (i.e. arteriosclerosis); decreased sensitivity; weakness; and
                     pregnancy.

Sitz Bath

- Description: A partial bath covering the pelvic region given in a specially designed tub. Historically, this procedure was a mainstay of hydrotherapy because of its ability to powerfully affect the organs of the lower abdomen and pelvis. It has fallen into disuse because of the labor-intensive nature of the treatment, inconvenience, and the fact that it is no longer taught in medical schools.

- Rationale: To increase circulation to the abdominal and pelvic organs. The Sitz bath provides direct effects corresponding to temperature and the length of time it is used: hot is stimulating and relaxing; cold increases the tone of smooth muscle; and neutral exerts a calming effect.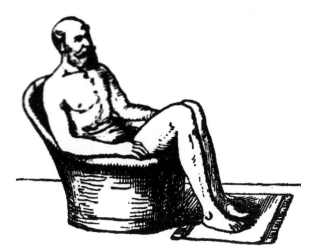

- Equipment: Sitz bath filled with water at the desired temperature; towels; sheet.

- Procedure: Help the patient sit in the tub. The water should come up over the hips to the abdomen. A sheet may be placed over the patient and the tub for privacy.

  Hot Sitz - Temperature of the water is 105 - 115 degrees F. and treatment time is from 2 - 10 minutes. Apply cold compress to the forehead.

  Cold Sitz - Temperature of the water is 55 - 75 degrees F. for a duration of 2 - 10 minutes.

Contrast Sitz - Alternating between hot and cold Sitz. Hot ranges from 105-115 degrees F and the cold 55-85 degrees F. The patient is treated in the hot Sitz bath for 3 minutes and transfers to the cold Sitz bath for 30 - 60 seconds. The procedure is repeated three times, always ending with cold. The water level in the hot tub is 1 inch higher than the cold. This bath is the most difficult to provide but has the most beneficial effects. Provide adequate draping to prevent chilling.

Neutral Sitz - Temperature of the water 92 - 97 degrees F. for a period of 15 minutes to 2 hours.

- Indications:

  Hot Sitz - acute and chronic cystitis; dysmenorrhea; chronic pelvic inflammatory disease; prostatitis; constipation; postpartum care; sciatica; painful hemorrhoids; congestive headache; skin problems in the pelvic area; after hemorrhoidectomy or cystoscopy surgeries. The hot Sitz is very analgesic and stimulating to pelvic circulation.

  Cold Sitz - increases the tone of smooth muscle of the uterus, bladder, and colon. It decreases the likelihood of bleeding from the uterus, lower bowel, and rectum. Indications: constipation; incontinence; menorrhagia; subinvolution of the uterus; enuresis; general tonic effect.

  Contrast Sitz - poor pelvic circulation and smooth muscle tone; vaginal infection; chronic pelvic inflammatory disease; chronic prostatitis; chronic constipation; postpartum care; hemorrhoids; fissures; congestive headache; following rectal surgery.

  Neutral Sitz - acute cystitis; pruritis; mental or sexual excitement; acute inflammation of prostate.

- Contraindications: General contraindications, as for other hot or cold treatments

Whirlpool Bath

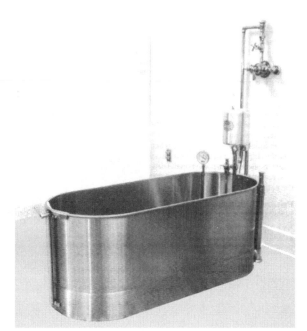

- **Description:** A partial immersion bath in which water is agitated and mixed with air, which is then directed against the affected area.

- **Rationale:** The pressure of the water against the body part will result in an increase in circulation to the area, as well as providing a cleansing mechanism.

- **Equipment:** Whirlpool bath with water either at a neutral or hot temperature; cold compress; towels; antiseptic.

- **Procedure:** Fill the whirlpool bath to desired height. Temperatures may range from neutral (94 - 97 degrees F.) to very hot (105 - 110 degrees). Add a teaspoon of antiseptic to the water. Remove any dressings covering a wound that the patient may have. Assist the patient into the bath. Apply a cold compress to the neck if very hot water is used. Circulate the agitated water over the area to be treated. Continue for 10 to 25 minutes. Assist the patient out of the bath. Dry him with a towel and allow time to rest.

- **Indications:** Poor circulation; muscle spasms and pain; wounds such as amputation stumps and burns; sprains and contusions after the first 36 hours; arthritis; fibrositis; post-operative orthopedic conditions; peripheral vascular disease; and peripheral nerve injuries - all are treated with neutral temperatures.

- **Contraindications:** Patient cannot tolerate the force of the water.

G. Irrigations & Miscellaneous External Applications

Nasal Irrigation

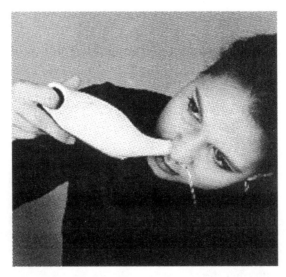

Neti Pot - Courtesy of Himalayan Institute Press

- Description: An infusion of water or medicated solution into the nose, which passes through the nasal passages and sinuses.

- Rationale: Nasal irrigations have been shown in numerous clinical trials to significantly reduce symptoms of paranasal disorders by washing away respiratory dust, pollen, and irritants; removing excess mucous; speeding healing of inflamed tissues; and restoring moisture and integrity to dry mucous membranes.

- Equipment: Neti Pot (as shown above), a commercial medical nasal irrigator, an irrigator attachment for Water Pik type devices, or a bulb syringe.

- Procedure: Fill the Neti pot with a solution of warm water and 1/4 tsp non-iodized salt (adding zinc, glycerin, or herbs as indicated), turn head to the side and insert Neti pot into upper nostril. Raise the Neti pot allowing the solution to flow into the nose, through the nasal passages and out the lower nostril. Repeat with other side.

- Indications: Acute or chronic upper respiratory infection, respiratory allergies, exposure to airborne pollutants, and dry mucous membranes.

- Contraindications: Undiagnosed respiratory conditions, children.

Enema

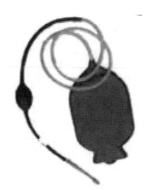

- **Description:** Insertion of plain water or water mixed with medical solutions into the rectum. There are many schools of thought regarding administering enemas. They are useful in cases of inflammation, congestion and /or pain anywhere in the body, especially when the bowels are not moving. The rectum has a reflex relationship throughout the body. Enemas should not be abused. They are remedial, not preventive.

- **Rationale:** An enema is used to cleanse the bowel and aid the body in eliminating toxins or infection. The temperature of the water used can help control blood flow to and from the abdomen and structures of the bowel. Enemas using hot water will encourage blood flow to the abdomen. Enemas using cold water decrease blood flow to the abdomen and encourage its flow to the legs, chest, and head.

- **Equipment:** Enema bag filled with water at the desired temperature and towels.

- **Procedure:** Fill the enema bag with water at the desired temperature. Ask the patient to lie on his back with the knees bent. Elevate the buttocks with a folded towel. Lubricate the nozzle of the enema bag with Vaseline and insert gently into the rectum toward the navel. Hold the bag above the patient and release the solution. After the patient holds as much solution as is practical, ask them to retain it for as long as possible, up to 15 - 20 minutes. Have the patient evacuate and rest.

- **Indications:** **Hot** - impacted feces; diarrhea; intestinal parasites; colitis. **Cold** – acute pelvic inflammatory disease; pelvic congestion; abdominal congestion. **Charcoal** - dissolve 1 - 5 tablespoons of charcoal in 2 quarts of water to be used for any toxic state such as drug ingestion, snakebite, or kidney failure. Also used for infections, inflamed fissures, and hemorrhoids.

- **Contraindications:** Diverticular disease, perforated colon, undiagnosed illness.

Colonic Irrigation

- **Description**
An infusion of water or medicated solution through the rectum, intended to fill the entire large intestine. The device for administering colonic irrigations has an inlet and outlet allowing the water or solution to enter and exit. Both temperature and pressure of colonic solution, as well as the vacuum, can be adjusted by the technician.

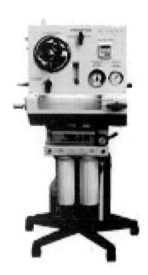

- **Rationale:** Colonics are administered to stimulate peristalsis, increase bile secretion, relieve flatus, increase muscle tone in a hypotonic colon, decrease muscle tone in a hypertonic colon, or to decrease autointoxication.

- **Equipment:** Colonic irrigation apparatus. Various commercial models are available.

- **Procedure:** This procedure requires specialized training and the patient should have a medical evaluation prior to beginning therapy.

- **Indications:** Chronic constipation due to hypotonic or hypertonic colon musculature, autointoxication due to chronically delayed transit time, chronic poor or incomplete digestion.

- **Contraindications:** Diverticular disease, perforated colon, gastrointestinal hemorrhage, ulcerations, hemorrhoids, severe cardiac disease, severe anemia, undiagnosed illness, and electrolyte imbalances. Untrained technician.

Vaginal Irrigation

- **Description:** A cleansing stream of water or medicated solution used internally by women for vaginal irrigation.

- **Rationale:** Douching is generally not necessary for women with normal vaginal secretions and is never recommended for pregnant women. Used to cleanse the area in vaginitis or cervicitis. Vinegar or Boric acid restore the normal vaginal pH (acid) and discourage growth of pathogenic organisms. Boric acid also exhibits antifungal properties. Yogurt or Acidophilus re-establish friendly flora, which compete with pathogens.

- **Equipment:** Irrigation (douche) kit or bulb syringe, vinegar (5%), boric acid, acidophilus or plain yogurt - unsweetened (with live cultures), bath tub or toilet.

- **Procedure:** Assemble the douche kit as per instructions. Fill it with 2 quarts of hot water from 105 to 110 degrees F. Sit or lie in a position of about a 45 degree angle. Insert the nozzle into the vagina and release the clasp to allow the solution to fill the area. Hold the tissue together around the nozzle for a more effective application. Hold the solution for approximately 15 seconds. Release the solution and repeat the procedure until all of the solution is used. For infections use 1 - 4 tablespoons of vinegar or one teaspoon of Boric acid to one quart of hot water. *Use this solution in the AM. Add contents of one Acidophilus capsule or 2 tablespoons of yogurt to *warm* water for use in the PM. Use vinegar and hot water only in postpartum care.

- **Indications:** Vaginitis; cervicitis; yeast infections; trichomoniasis; postpartum care.

- **Contraindications:** Bleeding, extreme vaginal irritation, conditions which have not responded within three days.

Poultice

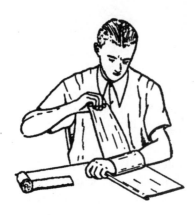

- **Description:** Defined as a hot or warm, moist, soft mass applied to the skin between two pieces of muslin, to soothe, relax, or stimulate aching or inflamed areas. The poultice should be large enough to cover a surface area twice as large as the area being treated. The substances used should absorb and hold water well.

- **Rationale:** Counter irritants, such as a mustard poultice, increase blood flow to tissue; hypertonic material such as clay and flaxseed cause the fluid in tissue to move to the skin's surface by the process of osmosis and reduce congestion and pain.

- **Equipment:** Various substances can be used that have medicinal properties. These substances include:

  Carrot - grate one or more carrots.

  Clay & Glycerin - the moist clay is further moistened with several drops of glycerin.

  Flaxseed - grind one tablespoon in a seed mill or blender and mix with one cup boiling water.

  Hops - fresh or dried leaves are moistened with hot water and then blended with a small amount of water to make a paste.

  Comfrey & Smartweed - fresh or dried leaves are moistened and blended with enough water to form a soft paste.

  Mustard - one tablespoon of dry mustard and four tablespoons of wheat flour are mixed (adult dosage); one tablespoon of dry mustard and eight tablespoons of wheat flour are mixed (child dosage); one tablespoon of dry mustard and twelve tablespoons of wheat flour are mixed (infant dosage). Add enough tepid water to make a thin paste that can be spread.

- Equipment:
  Large mixing bowl, metal tray or platter.
  Blender or seed mill.
  Plastic, muslin, cotton cloth, gauze, or paper towel.
  Alcohol or mineral oil.
  Ace bandage, towel, pins (to hold poultice).
  Sponge or washcloth.

- Procedure:
  Clay - Apply clay paste directly to skin surface. Cover with several layers of cotton cloth or gauze. Keep poultice moist for 6-10 hr., applying water as needed. Rinse thoroughly and dry. Wait 1-2 hr. and re-apply moist dressing.

  Carrot, Flaxseed, Hops, Comfrey & Smartweed - Take paper towel and spread mixture on towel. The mixture is then laid directly on the skin. Cover with a plastic sheet that extends one inch over the edges on all sides. Hold in place with ace bandage. Leave poultice on 30 minutes to 8 hours. Remove and sponge the surface clean. Friction massage the area with alcohol. Dry thoroughly.

  Mustard - Warm a large platter or metal tray. Place the cloth on the heated tray or platter and spread the mixture from the center of the tray outward to the edges (leave a margin wide enough to lap over sides of area being treated). When the patient is ready, remove the poultice from the tray. Place one thin layer of cotton cloth between the patient's skin and the mustard paste. Cover the area with a plastic sheet. Place towel (folded or flat) and pin to hold poultice in place. Leave the poultice on 20 minutes. **Caution**: if the patient complains of stinging or burning, or if the skin becomes **extremely** red, remove the poultice. Wipe area with cloth dipped in mineral oil to remove all mustard traces. Cover area with towel and pin in place. Cover with a snug fitting sweater or cotton shirt. Leave on all night.

- Indications:
  Pneumonia, peritonitis and other deep-seated inflammations, arthritic joints, back aches, muscle spasm, congestion, abscesses, crusted lesions, and inflammatory skin diseases.

- Contraindications: Skin sensitivity, open wounds and debilitated individuals (special attention). Mustard can cause blistering or ulceration and appropriate precautions must be taken. Also, the poultice can encourage bacterial growth--if pus increases, discontinue.

Shirodhara

- **Description:** Traditional Ayurvedic treatment wherein a small stream of warm sesame oil is allowed to gently pour onto the forehead of the reclining patient.

- **Rationale:** The warm temperature and steady flow of the oil are relaxing. In Ayurvedic terms, Shirodhara is considered to be a cooling treatment: balancing the Vata dosha, nourishing the nervous system, stabilizing the mind, and increasing the glow of complexion.

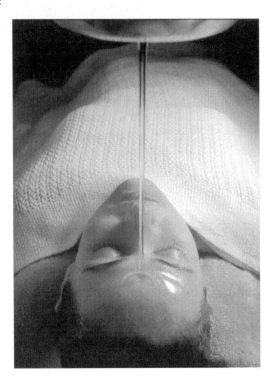

- **Equipment:** Bowl or funnel with spigot to control the flow of oil creating a small stream which is applied to the forehead of the patient. A receptacle for collecting the oil as it pours over the patient's head. A stand to hold the bowl greatly facilitates the procedure. At least 1 quart of suitable oil, usually high quality sesame oil is used.

- **Procedure:** Fill the Shirodhara bowl with the warm sesame oil. Extend the patient's head and neck slightly to insure the oil runs over the head and not into the eyes. Open the spigot and adjust the flow to allow a small stream of warm oil to gently pour onto the forehead of the reclining patient. Continue to collect oil in receptacle and return to the Shirodhara bowl. The treatment should last from 30 to 60 minutes. Allow the patient to rest.

- **Indications:** Insomnia, tension, anxiety, prior to massage or other treatments.

- **Contraindications:** Undiagnosed illness, sensitivity to oil.

Aquatic Exercise Therapy

- **Description:** Aquatic Exercise Therapy is the union of aquatic exercise and physical therapy.

- **Rationale:** Buoyancy relieves stress on weight-bearing joints and permits movement to be accomplished without the opposing effects of gravity. A patient submersed to their neck off-loads approximately 90% of their body weight. The warm temperature of the water brings about positive physiological changes. Water provides more resistance than air.

- **Equipment:** Exercise or swimming pool with water temperature ranging from 89 to 96° F. Ambient air temperature should be slightly lower than that of the water to allow cool down following therapy.

- **Procedure:** Aquatic exercise therapy includes specific exercise programs for the rehabilitation of various conditions. Each exercise program is organized into four specific components: warm-up, stretching, muscular strength, and endurance training and relaxation. Massage, traction, floatation, and resistance devices, and therapeutic breathing techniques may be incorporated. Water temperature and depth as well as each individual patient's diagnosis, limitations and goals, should be considered in treatment design.

- **Indications:** Pain and muscle spasm, decreased ROM, muscle atrophy, post surgery and post stroke neuromuscular reeducation, functional training, and maintenance of posture, balance, and coordination.

- **Contraindications:** Undiagnosed illness, communicable disease.

Watsu

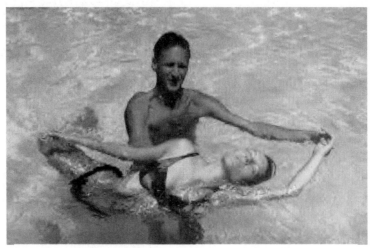

Watsu - Courtesy of Tal Hurley, The Watsu Oasis

- Description: Watsu is a form of aquatic bodywork developed by Harold Dull at Harbin Hot Springs (CA) in the early eighties and combines elements of Zen shiatsu, Swedish massage, movement therapy, and hydrotherapy.

- Rationale: Buoyancy relieves stress on weight-bearing joints and permits movement to be accomplished without the opposing effects of gravity. The warm temperature of the water brings about positive physiological and psychological changes. The holding or "cradling" by the water and therapist encourage trust and deep relaxation. Watsu is considered to be a somatic therapy, although many therapists speak of energetic and emotional benefits.

- Equipment: Exercise or swimming pool with water temperature of 94 to 98° F.

- Procedure: Watsu begins with warm water. The therapist holds or cradles the patient, supporting their head, neck, and legs. Gentle swaying and rocking help the patient to relax. The patient is then floated thru a variety of positions while the therapist massages, stretches, and applies pressure to specific acupressure points.

- Indications: Tension, anxiety, insomnia, stress, pain and muscle spasm, decreased ROM, post stroke neuromuscular reeducation, and for the maintenance of posture, balance and coordination.

- Contraindications: Undiagnosed illness, communicable disease.

Liquid Sound

- **Description:**

  Liquid Sound is a form of aquatic therapy recently developed at Bad Sulza, Germany. It combines the high-tech elements of color therapy, sound therapy, movement, and bodywork therapy with more traditional balneotherapy.

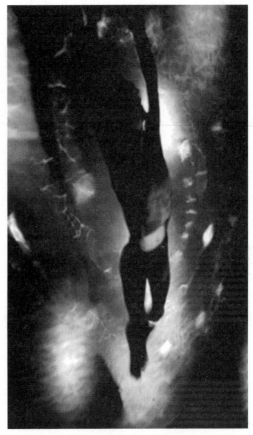

Courtesy of Liquid Sound - Bad Sulza

- **Rationale:**

  The increased buoyancy of hypertonic saline spring water relieves the stress on weight-bearing joints and permits floating or movement to be accomplished without the opposing effects of gravity. The warm (94-98 ° F) temperature of the water brings about positive physiological and psychological changes. The support of the water and the therapist encourages deep relaxation. Both sound and pulsed colored light are introduced via the water medium.

- **Equipment:**

  Exercise or swimming pool with water temperature of 94 to 98° F. Color and sound generating equipment.

- **Procedure:**

  Patients may float unattended in the pool, experiencing both water mediated light and sound, or be guided through a prescribed series of stretches and movements by an aquatic therapist.

- **Indications:**

  Tension, anxiety, insomnia, stress, pain, and muscle spasm, decreased ROM, chronic fatigue, fibromyalgia, post stroke/surgery neuromuscular reeducation, maintenance of posture, balance, and coordination, pulmonary disorders, chronic dermatological conditions, and disorders of psychosomatic origin.

- **Contraindications:** Undiagnosed illness, communicable disease.

Aqua PT

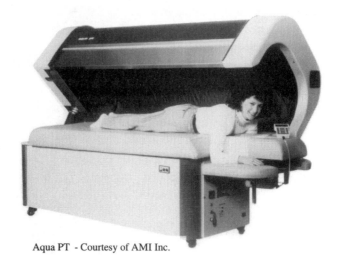

Aqua PT - Courtesy of AMI Inc.

- Description: The Aqua PT machine is described as providing "Dry Hydrotherapy." It is a self contained, bed-like device, which is blanketed by a waterproof barrier and an acrylic top canopy that closes over the patient. The canopy contains 36 traveling water jets capable of producing 2-11 pounds of force at 2-10 cycles per second.

- Rationale: Mechanical massage effects result from the pressure of the 36 water jets moving over the body. Sustained thermal effects result from the dry heat produced inside the capsule. Water temperature is adjustable from 90-104° F. Pressure, travel speed, and pulsation rates are also controllable. The patient can control some parameters during the treatment via a hand-held panel.

- Equipment: Aqua PT machine (18 gallons of water - self contained).

- Procedure: Open canopy and help patient to recline on cushion in either prone or supine position. Set treatment parameters and initiate the treatment cycle. Treatment time is typically 10 to 20 minutes.

- Indications: Fibromyalgia, RSD, *chronic and myofascial pain, muscle spasm, decreased ROM, prior to manual therapy.

- Contraindications: Undiagnosed illness, acute trauma, and communicable disease.

   *Recent research from the University of Miami, Pain & Rehabilitation Center supports the use of the Aqua PT in patients with these conditions.

IX. SPA TECHNIQUES & PROCEDURES

A. Introduction

The development of spa therapies has evolved from the consumer's desire for alternative treatments for relaxation, renewal, and rejuvenation. As stress and stress-related illnesses increasingly impact the nation's productivity and health care, alternative ways of "de-stressing" are in demand. This evolution provides therapies that were only available in European spas or up-scale "destination" spa retreats. As the American public experiences spa therapies and becomes educated in their benefits, the demand continues to increase. The industry (care providers) must keep up with advanced body-therapy and hydrotherapy treatments to provide the services and benefits demanded.

European spas are generally four weeks in duration. Guests are seen by a physician and examined. The physician prescribes a daily program. The guest usually experiences what is termed a "bath (cure) reaction." After the initial treatment, the guest feels better. Symptoms may then be exacerbated, leaving the guest feeling worse. In the fourth week, there should be a distinct improvement, which is retained over a long period of time.

The American spa industry has experienced a slow revival from the 1950s to present. In the 1950s and '60s, spas were primarily devoted to weight loss. By the 1970s and '80s, programs were offered for diet, exercise, body, and mind. Now in the 1990s, the public is demanding many varied services ranging from "destination" spas to "day" spas.

Organizations such as Club Spa USA-The Day Spa Association, and conferences, such as those sponsored by the International Spa & Fitness Association, have been formed to develop, promote, and educate the industry. As the interest in day-spas grows, more products, equipment, and advanced training providers appear.

Spa development seems to be dividing into two avenues, one associated with the extension of "full service salons" and the other with holistic day-spas, which offer more therapeutic treatments. It is essential that therapists receive specialized training and be properly licensed before offering these specialized treatments. Disenchantment with some current drug therapies, as well as medical conditions which do not seem to respond to the mainstream medical treatments, result in people seeking "refuge" and "hope" at spa treatment facilities.

The spa treatments contained in this text are some of those more commonly utilized. New treatments, recipes, and menus are constantly being developed in this field. *The author has diligently searched the current literature regarding the following "spa" therapies and has found a dearth of scientific evidence to support many of the claims made for these treatments.* He has however, attempted to describe the treatments contained herein from a rational and scientific point of view, despite the lack of published empirical data. These treatments fall into broad categories defined as Balneotherapy, Peloid baths, Showers, Water Massage and Aromatherapy.

B. Balneotherapy

Balneotherapy is the systematic application of mineral water for therapeutic purposes. There is a broad range of opinion regarding the effectiveness of one spa treatment over the other. Little scientific evidence exists. Early analysis of mineral waters attached importance to certain elements such as anions (iron, sulfur), cations (iodine), and trace elements. As we entered the 20th Century, spa physicians began to see Balneotherapy as part of a total treatment, including diet, exercise, stress management, hydrotherapeutic baths and rest.

There are nine distinct groups of dominant or active ions in water. They are as follows:

Chloride	Chloride ions prevail.
Sulfur	Alkaline or hydrogen sulfide.
Sulfate	Sulfate, sodium and magnesium.
Acid	Hydrogen ion concentration containing sulfate or chloride ions - pH is less then 7.
Iron	Ferrous iron, bicarbonate, and an excess of carbon dioxide.
Alkaline	pH is more than 8 with bicarbonate & sodium.
Calcium	Calcium and bicarbonate with an excess of carbon dioxide, sulfate or chloride.
Rare elements	Arsenic, lithium, bromine, and iodine.
Other	Water with low mineral content.

Mineral waters are also classified by their medical indications. They are:

Alkalizing waters	Predominantly ions of sodium, calcium, and bicarbonate.
Stimulating	Rich in ions of sodium, chloride and sulfate.
Stimulating & alkalizing	Large amounts of ions of sodium, calcium, bicarbonate, and chloride.
Diuretic	Low mineral content and are hypotonic with calcium and sulfate ions.
Diuretic & stimulating	High content of sodium, calcium, chloride, and sulfate ions.
Reconstituent	Contains ferrous ions.
Anticatarrhal	Charged with hydrogen sodium sulfide.
Energetic	Poorly mineralized and hyperthermic.
Peloids	Used as local applications or full baths, solids (moor, peat, and thermal mud) mixed with hot water.

Thermal and hyperthermal springs have been used for centuries. There are only two groups of springs whose chemical content is of special (medicinal) value--sulfur waters and hypertonic chloride waters, and only when they are also thermal or hyperthermal should they be considered medicinal.

C. Peloids

Peloids are defined as substances, which originate in nature by biological and geological processes. In a finely divided state, they are mixed with water and applied as baths and packs for medical purposes. Peloids are often used as packs or in baths, alternating with thermal waters. However, some spas apply pelotherapy exclusively. Peloids vary greatly in composition but fall into general categories:

- Peat (spagnosum).
- Moor (uliginorum).
- Earthy moor (terra uliginosa).
- Muds (limus).

Peats consist mostly of spagnum or bog moss; composed of organic matter and plant debris, their reaction is acid. Moors consist mostly of reed, sedge, molinientalia, and alnion; mainly organic, but when mixed with mineral waters, their reaction is acid. Earthy moors consist of mixtures of moors containing vegetable and inorganic components and mud, with a considerable amount of lime, and are acid or subneutral. The inorganic components of mud consist of finely disintegrated rock and algae component.

Techniques

Spa therapy is only a part of the total overall therapeutic plan and does not replace the patient's medical care. Spas "cures" are usually at least four weeks in duration, but may extend to seven weeks. Shorter periods of time are usually unrewarding. Spa therapies are complex procedures, which have thermal, chemical, medicinal, and psychological affects on the body.

The general condition of the patient determines the number, duration, and temperature of the baths. Baths can be alternated with peloid treatments. There should be at least one day of rest between treatments. Patients are referred by national health plans. These spas employ highly trained staff, including massage therapists and physical therapists. They also are equipped with all the necessary hydrotherapy paraphernalia.

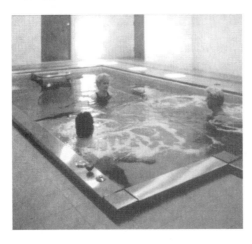

Many of the hydrotherapy techniques have been previously discussed. However, some of these techniques have been modified and are commonly used in "spa" treatments. The following are some of the most commonly used.

D. Massage

Underwater Pressure Massage (Hydro Tub)

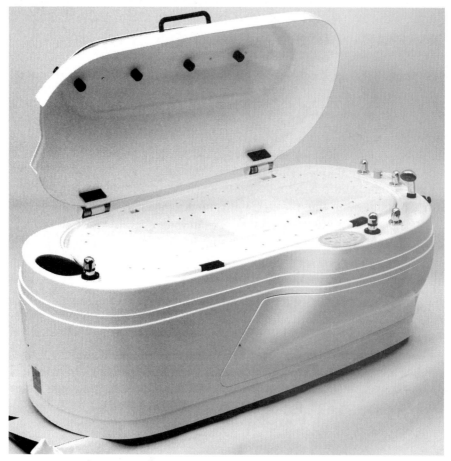

Aromatherm Hydro Tub - Courtesy of Cosmopro

- Description: A hose delivers water to the body, under varying degrees of
  pressure, in a systematic procedure while the body is submerged in
  a tub of water.

- Rationale: The temperature of the water and the varying force stimulates
  the circulation and relaxes muscles and organs.

- Equipment: Tub of warm water. An internal pump draws the water needed
  for the massage from the tub of water and returns it under pressure. The water pump is noiseless, enclosed in plastic casing, and
  can convey up to 200 liter/minute. The pressure ranges from 0.5 to
  a maximum of 7.0 bar absolute pressure units. The hose has a
  number of interchangeable nozzles.

The tub is made of reinforced fiber, polyester-resin casting, tempered to provide heat and shock resistance.

- Procedure:

The temperature of the water in the tub ranges from 96.8 F to l00.4 F. The temperature of the water under pressure can be adjusted, and is precisely measured by a built-in thermometer.

The massage lasts from 20-30 minutes.

The pressure is controlled by a manometer or pressure gauge. Adjustments can be made because the pressure measured by the manometer will be higher than when applied to the body, as the pressurized water has to travel through the water that is already in the tub before it reaches the client. Nozzles are usually medium to large in size (smaller ones can cause stabbing pain, and force the muscles to react defensively). The massage is individualized. Body builders and athletes with large muscle mass can withstand a greater water pressure than clients with sensitive tissue. Those with larger muscle mass could begin at 2.0-4.0 bar and slowly increase the pressure. For clients with sensitive tissue, begin at 0.5-1.5 bar and raise the pressure slowly to determine the tolerance level.

The client rests in a supine position for a few minutes to become accustomed to the water. The client then turns to a side-lying position. Begin with the client on his/her left side. Massage the right side of the back area and then ask the client to turn on his/her right side and complete the left side of the body. The massage is delivered in varying treatment positions. The strokes follow a caudal-cranial direction and are slow. Long diagonal strokes, or smaller circular patterns, are used on large muscle groups. Small circular strokes and long, slightly curved strokes are used for small, long-slim muscle groups and intercostals.

Sensitive areas of the body, such as the spinous processes, bone spurs, genitalia, anus, back of the knees, and female breasts and axillary area are the be avoided.

Back & Pelvis: The client lies on his/her side, the hips and knees are slightly bent, and the head and neck are supported. Direct the stream of water to the thoracolumbar fascia; the gluteals; lumbar region between iliac crest and lower ribcage; spinous process (medial) to latissimus dorsi (lateral); the lower thorax to cervical segment at the inferior angle of the scapula; the spinous process to the latissimus dorsi and the intercostals; the inferior

130

angle of the scapula to the subocciptal triangle, including teres major and minor. The muscles of the back, the erector spinae, latissimus dorsi, and trapezius are massaged with a diagonal or circular motion. Circular and diagonal motion is also suitable for the neck, trapezius, rhomboids, and scapular area.

Arms: Direct pressure caudal to cranial from dorsal side of hands upward toward and including the deltoids.

Legs: Direct pressure caudal to cranial from calcaneous, including gastrocnemius, soleus, and hamstrings (medial to lateral).

Anterior Neck and Thoracic Wall: The client is supine. Direct the stream of water from the anterior aspect of the neck between clavicular muscles; thoracic wall, including pectoral muscles; intercostal muscles; and lateral aspects of latissimus dorsi. The intercostal area should be stroked out from the spinal column to the sternum. The large thoracic muscles and pectoralis major are massaged with a gentle circulating stream.

Abdomen: The abdominal region is massaged with a gentle circular stream, which follows the course of the large intestine.

Arms & Legs: Repeat massage of anterior arms. Begin at palmar surface and move superior to biceps. Begin legs at malleolus and move superior, working anterior and lateral lower leg muscles; work quadriceps superior from patella to below the inguinal area, working medial to lateral.

If desired, a cold affusion is applied to stimulate circulation. The client rests for 30 minutes.

- Indications: Fractures, osteosyntheses, dislocations, sprains, subacute contusions, sciatica, lumbago, brachialgia, joint and scar contractures, myogeloses, degenerative spinal disorders, chronic joint rheumatism, muscular rheumatism, ankylosing spondylitis, scoliosis, flaccid and spastic paralyses, muscular hypertonicity, and post event or post strenuous training of athletes.

- Contraindications: Recent athletic injuries, open wounds, acute hematomas, acute muscle, ligament and tendon conditions and recent fractures, cardiovascular insufficiencies, venous disorders, thromboses, and varicosities.

© Pine Island Publishers Inc. 2003

Stone Massage

- **Description:** Treatment utilizing heated or cooled stones; which are used as massage tools, or solely for their thermal and energetic effects.

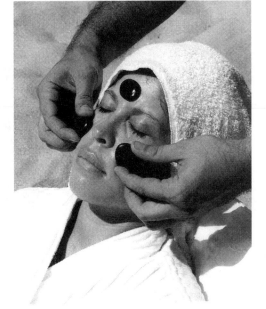

Stone Facial - Courtesy of T.H. Stone

- **Rationale:** Stones are used to conduct heat or cold. Sedimentary stones are used with oil as massage tools to administer effleurage or deep trigger point therapy. Stones may be placed upon acupressure points to either stimulate or sedate. Semi-precious stones are placed over corresponding Chakras.

- **Equipment:** Smooth river rocks or stones -- basalt is commonly used for heat. Semi-precious stones (amethyst, sodalite, turquoise, rose quartz, tigers eye, jasper and bloodstone) for use over Chakras. A heating and/or cooling unit. Thermometer, massage oil, towels, blanket, and sanitizing solution.

- **Procedure:** Heat stones to 120-125° F. Cool stones to 32° F. Apply oil to patient if performing massage. Choose stones based upon the patients condition and needs -- hot to increases circulation and soften tissue, cold to decrease circulation and tone tissue. Sanitize stones after use.

- **Indications:** Heated stones -- hypertonic muscles, acupressure points needing stimulation, and prior to deep tissue manual massage. Cooled stones -- inflammation, acupressure points needing sedation, and in deep tissue trigger point massage.

- **Contraindications:** Same as for other heat or cold therapies. Marble is not recommended, as it is very cold and can damage tissue.

E. Baths

Peloid Bath

- Description:

Peloids are administered as a semi-fluid poultice or full-body bath. Peloids are gentler than water at the same temperature because of their specific heat. Peloids are poorer heat conductors than water.

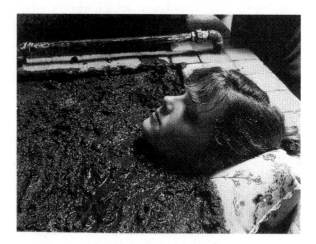

Full Body Peloid Bath

Because the first layer of peloid mass forms an isolating barrier around the body surface, further heat is transmitted to the body through this barrier. Because of this property, higher temperatures can be used, and the heat is transmitted to the body in a uniform and steady manner. The point of thermal indifference (tepid bath) is 93 F for water, but 100.4 F for peloids.

- Rationale:

Peloid applications produce hyperemia and hyperthermia if followed by a full dry blanket pack. Systemic temperature and respiratory rates increase, as well as pulse rates. Blood pressure falls. Dilatation of peripheral vessels occurs; hyperemia increases cell metabolism; heat exerts an analgesic and spasmolytic affect. Sulfurs and incompletely oxidized compounds such as hydrogen sulfide, alkaline sulfide, and polysulfides can be reabsorbed into the chondroitin sulfate of the articular cartilage. Estrogenic substances may be absorbed through the skin and may account for why peloids help in degenerative arthritis. A series of peloid baths is a stress, which may act strongly on the pituitary-adrenal system. The chemical composition is secondary since most of the compounds cannot penetrate the skin.

- **Equipment:**   Bath tub, various peloids can be used for whatever the desired outcome; the properties of the peloids has been discussed.

- **Procedure:**   Tub filled with peloid combination.
  Client lies in tub covered with mixture. Temperature is maintained at l07.6 degrees F and bath lasts for no longer than 25 minutes. After a peloid bath, and more so with a full blanket wrap, profuse sweating occurs. Be cautious of dehydration. The client can loose up to 1.5 liters of water through perspiration. Provide adequate water for hydration during and after bath.

- **Indications:**   The most important indications are inflammatory and degenerative disorders of the loco-motor system. Rheumatoid arthritis patients are most often referred for spa therapy as well as those with Ankylosing spondylitis, joint deformities, psoriatic arthropathy (benefits most with large amounts of hydrogen or sulfides), infective arthritis (only after the acute signs and symptoms have been absent for three months), and degenerated articular cartilage. Healing is unlikely, but thermal sulfur waters seem to benefit--probably from the soothing of the synovial membrane by massage, and systematic exercises, rather than the sulfur.

- **Contraindications:** Inflammatory joint diseases, acute rheumatic diseases, and special attention to the overall condition of elderly patients, who often have arteriosclerosis and myocardial disease.

Fango Salicyl Mud Bath

- **Description:** Mud bath consisting of fango – pure volcanic ash, salicyl (aspirin) powder and pine needle extract.

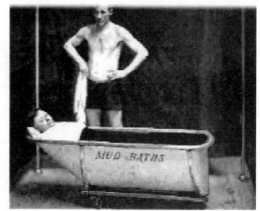

Fango Salicyl Mud Bath
Battlecreek Sanitarium - Circa 1925

- **Rationale:** The volcanic ash helps cleanse and exfoliate the skin. It replenishes minerals and the heat created promotes relaxation. The pine needle extract stimulates blood circulation, while the salicyl (aspirin) acts as a pain reliever.

- **Equipment:** Tub, water, Fango-Pine extract, Salicyl mix, Towels.

- **Procedure:** Mix 2 ounces of fango salicyl product with 4 cups warm water in tub.
Swirl to dissolve.
Add warm (102 degrees F) water.
Submerge client in bath for 10-20 minutes.
Have client shower with cool or cold water.
Wrap him in a warm blanket and advise rest for 10-20 minutes.

- **Indications:** Dry skin, muscle spasms.

- **Contraindications:** Hypersensitivity to Aromatic herbs/oils or salicylates.

Milk Whey Bath

- **Description:** Warm water bath with milk whey additive to restore acidity to the skin.

- **Rationale:** Milk whey is a natural cleanser and moisturizer, helping to retain and replenish the skin's protective acid (5.5 pH) nature.

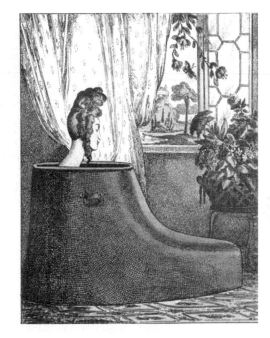

Sabotiéres or Shoe-shaped bathtub - Circa 1750

- **Equipment:** Tub with warm water; Milk whey; Towel/blanket.

- **Procedure:** Mix 2 ounces of milk whey with 4 cups warm water in tub.
Add warm water (102 degrees F) to tub & fill.
Submerge client in bath for 10-20 minutes.
Wrap him in a warm blanket and advise rest for 10-20 minutes.

- **Indications:** Damaged, dry, sensitive skin.

- **Contraindications:** Hypersensitivity to dairy products.

Hot Mineral Water Bath

- **Description:** Balneotherapy is the systematic application of mineral water for therapeutic purposes. Historically, users sit or recline in hot / warm mineral pools.

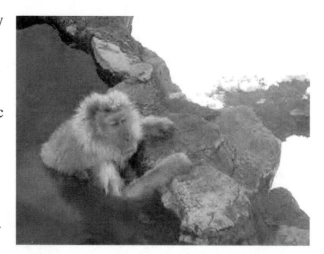

Monkey Bathing in Hot Mineral Springs at Nagano, Japan

- **Rationale:** Used when an increase in metabolism and circulation is needed. The resulting dilation of blood vessels increases blood flow and produces tissue relaxation. Also with an increase in metabolism, there is an increase in body temperature causing sweating and encouraging an elimination of metabolic byproducts. There is no heat lost in this procedure due to 100% humidity.

- **Equipment:** Hot springs or mineral pool, tub with hot mineral water.

- **Procedure:** Recline or sit in pool or bath for 10 to 15 minutes (but not longer than 25 minutes). Provide adequate water for hydration during and after bath. Follow with cool bath or spray for tonic effect.

- **Indications:** Musculoskeletal pain, stiffness of joints, Rheumatoid Arthritis, certain dermatological conditions, general relaxation, or in preparation for massage.

- **Contraindications:** Hypertension; diabetes; anemia; heart disease; peripheral vascular disease (i.e. arteriosclerosis); decreased sensitivity; weakness; and pregnancy.

Floatation or Sensory Deprivation Tank

- **Description:** Floating of the body in a shallow tub or tank of hypertonic water at neutral temperature (94 to 98 degrees F). in an area which is generally dark and quiet.

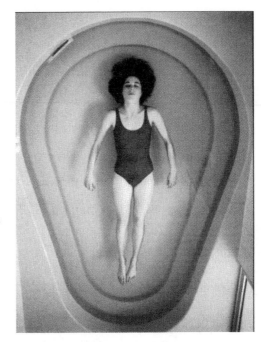

- **Rationale:** The neutral temperature, relative weightlessness, darkness, and quiet serve to diminish CNS activity to produce a relaxing, yet aware state.

Floatation Tank - Courtesy of ALAR

- **Equipment:** Isolation tank with water at 94 -98 degrees F, salt (a typical 300 gallon tank would require 1,200 lbs of Epson salts), heater, pump, and filtration system. Towels.

- **Procedure:** Assist the patient into the tank. Allow the patient to lie quietly and relax. Music may be used when appropriate. A session may last from 45 to 60 minutes, or longer, for conditions such as insomnia. Stay with the patient for the duration of treatment. Assist the patient out of the tub and dry gently. Offer water to hydrate and allow him to rest.

- **Indications:** Insomnia; irritability; anxiety; depression; for accelerated learning and visualization; fever; acute high blood pressure; peripheral edema; drug/alcohol withdrawal; pregnancy toxemia; chronic pain; dermatosis.

- **Contraindications:** Skin conditions aggravated by water such as eczema; serious cardiac weakness.

F. Aromatherapy

> "He is happiest who hath power to gather wisdom from a flower"
> Mary Howitt, c. 1825

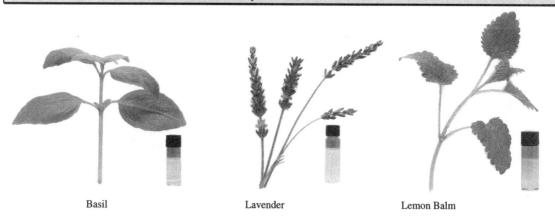

Basil   Lavender   Lemon Balm

Aromatherapy is a science and art that uses natural fragrant essential oils, herbs, and plant extracts to aid good health and beauty. These oils have been used throughout centuries, from the time of the Pharaohs, to promote health, beauty and enhance a sense of wellbeing. They are used in baths, saunas, and massages as well as fragrance dispensers.

> "Excellent herbs had our fathers of old,
> Excellent herbs to ease their pain,
> Alexanders and Marigold, Eyebright, Orris and Elecampane."
> *Rudyard Kipling*

The following is a recipe for eye inflammation translated from hieroglyphics of Egyptian physicians: Myrrh, "Great Protectors" seed, Copper oxide, Lemon pips, Northern cypress flowers, Antimony, Gazelle's droppings, Onyx offal and White oil. Place in water, let stand for one night, strain through a cloth, and smear over the eye for four days. Myrrh is still used today as an anti-inflammatory agent.

These essential oils are fragrant, volatile extracts from flowers, leaves, spices, fruits, woods, and roots. They are highly concentrated and contain vitamins, hormones, antibiotics, and antiseptics. Their chemistry generally contains alcohols, esters, ketones, aldehydes, and terpenes. The odoriferous materials are formed in the chloroplasts of the leaf. Here they combine with glucose to form glucosides. They are soluble in alcohol, ether, and fixed oils (but insoluble in water). The essences are extracted by distillation.

> "God in his infinite goodness and bounty hath by the medium of Plants,
> bestowed almost all food, clothing and medicine upon man."—
> Gerarde's *Herbal* (1636).

Aromatherapy is believed to use the sense of smell to affect the portions of the brain, which control mood. These scents may influence the emotions; and relax or stimulate the body, mind, and spirit. The oils penetrate the skin during warm baths and massage. The use of clove oil for a toothache, peppermint oil for indigestion, and eucalyptus for inhalations is well known. Specific aromatherapy bath treatments follow this discussion. The aroma, as well as the contact with the skin, relax, stimulate, and improve circulation. Aromatherapy can be applied in perfumes, steams, baths, massages, compresses, and diffusers.

Essential oils affect the body's physiological processes (stimulant, relaxant, spasmolytic, anti-infective), acting on the skin (topically - moisturizing, dehydrating or stimulating) and the psyche (soul), causing mental, emotional, and behavioral changes. Synergies are blends of certain essential oils that enhance the benefits of the separate oils. Aromasols are water-soluble versions of essential oil synergies, and are used when water solubility is desired such as body wraps, compresses, facial steaming, and manual lymphatic drainage. The varied uses of aromatherapy include environmental fragrancing, skin and body care products, and baths.

Currently, there are a number of educational mediums available--videos, books, and practical reference posters. Seminars are also available offering certification courses in aromatherapy. It is imperative that the therapist understands the botanical and clinical aspects of the 80+ different essential oils when blending and using these oils in spa treatments and massage. Knowledge of the exact dilution of the oils, what medium to use, the length of the treatment, as well as the indications and contraindications, is of utmost importance to insure the client's wellbeing and enhance the results of the treatment.

Robert Tisserand's, *The Art of Aromatherapy,* describes the applications and effects of various oils on the body systems. They are:

- **Digestive System**

  Oils may be given orally; by enemas or spinal massage, especially over dorsal and lumbar areas, and compresses over the stomach area or abdomen.

  Increases peristalsis--useful for constipation, flatulence, and lack of intestinal tone. It is not known if the oils act via the nervous system or have a direct effect. Camphor, cinnamon, fennel, marjoram, and rosemary are commonly used.

  Reduces smooth muscle spasm--Thyme counteracts adrenaline spasm; Melissa, sage, and thyme reduce acetylcholine spasm; clove, black pepper, and cinnamon leaf counteract stomach acidity by raising the pH of gastric juice.

[handwritten note: Does not need to be oil. Sometimes the herbs themselves]

140

- **Lymphatic System**

An American study completed in 1958 concluded that essential oils were more effective against bacteria when used undiluted and not blended with other oils. None were effective when infused. Cinnamon, eucalyptus, and oreganum were the most effective. Lavender proved to be the most effective in stimulating the immune system and increasing white blood corpuscles. Chamomile, lemon, thyme, pine needle, sandalwood, and vetivert are thought to increase leukocytosis. Bergamot and lemon have also shown to be effective immune system stimulants. The effect occurs whether taken orally, inhaled, or through cutaneous absorption.

- **Respiratory System**

May be given orally, inhaled, or by spinal massage--especially to the cervical or dorsal area or by compresses. The antiseptic, antispasmodic, and expectorant actions of these oils are of interest. Antiseptics such as bergamot, cinnamon, and eucalyptus are most valuable. Bergamot oil is effective against the diphtheria bacillus; garlic oil and camphor oil have been successful in pneumonia; cinnamon, eucalyptus, or black pepper are useful with some types of influenza. The antispasmodic effect is thought to be direct. Clary, fennel, peppermint, rose, and thyme at a concentration of 50-100 y/ml are effective antispasmodics. Camphor, as well as eucalyptus and lemon, are general respiratory stimulants.

- **Urinary System**

Treatments are given orally or via baths, lumbo-sacral massage, or local compresses. Juniper, sage, sandalwood and thyme are effective against urinary tract infection with staphylococcus aureus. These oils as well as camphor are good diuretics. Juniper enhances glomerular filtration and produces an increase in the amounts of potassium, sodium, and chlorine excretion. Chamomile and geranium have been used to dissolve urinary stones.

- **Reproductive System**

Oils are used orally, applied in compresses to the lower abdomen, in baths, some vaginal douches, and in massage to the lower back. A study conducted in 1930 found bergamot oil effective against gonococcus in a dilution of 1:600. Sandalwood is useful in treating gonorrhea.

Oils of Pennyroyal and savin are highly toxic. However, when applied externally or in relatively small doses, they have a emmenagogic affect (increased menstruation). Oils such as jasmine and juniper induce labor by stimulating uterine contractions.

Some oils are reputed to be aphrodisiacs, but there are no conclusive studies. Jasmine and ylang-ylang are two such notable oils.

- **Endocrine System**

Oils may stimulate glands to increase hormonal secretions or they may act as quasi-hormones themselves. Basil, geranium, pine, rosemary, jasmine, and sage are adrenal cortex stimulants. Phytohormones are substances found in plants that chemically resemble animal hormones. They are found in pollen extracts, eucalyptus, fennel, hops, dandelion, garlic, licorice root, sarsaparilla, ginseng, and many other plants. Estrogenic activity may be increased by aniseed, fennel, and eucalyptus.

- **Nervous System**

Stimulating oils are cedar, cardamom, fennel, cinnamon, lemon, peppermint, and ylang-ylang. These oils are useful in treating states of depression, languor and disorders associated with lack of nerve function such as paralysis, loss of voice, and conditions of "coldness." Rosemary is used for loss of memory and inability to concentrate.

Sedating oils are used for hysteria, insomnia, and certain states of nervousness. Lavender and Melissa have been shown to have pronounced sedative actions. Stupefying oils include Melissa, thyme and peppermint in large doses. Calamus, clary sage, and lavender have some anti-convulsive properties.

Convulsive oils include rosemary, fennel, hyssop, sage (not clary), and wormwood. Nutmeg oil is highly convulsive and should never be taken by epileptics.

> "My father took down some bottles from over the fireplace & mixed several liquids in a bowl. He then made a compress by folding a small piece of flannel, soaked it in the liquid and placed it on the man's side. Within half an hour the pains had gone and his face was no longer screwed up out of all recognition as it had been. Gripping the table in my excitement I couldn't take my eyes off him: it was a miracle!
> "Papa, did *you do that!*"
> "Mon cheri, he who causes the plants to grow is the one who did it."
> *Of Men and Plants*--Maurice Messegue

Aromatherapy Baths

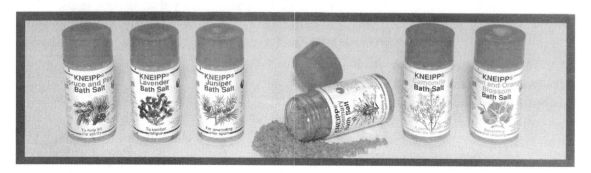

Herbal Bath Salts - Courtesy of Kneipp Corporation of America

- **Description:** Essential oils and bath salts are mixed with bath water to create the desired outcome or effects. Some are listed separately following this general section on aromatherapy baths.

- **Rational:** Stimulates or sedates physiological processes.

- **Equipment:** Tub of warm water
  Essential oil(s) or herbal bath salts of choice

- **Procedure:** 2 ounces of herbal bath salts are used per bath.
  Temperature is 96 F.
  Duration is 15-20 minutes
  Followed by 15-20 minutes of rest.

- **Indications:** See the following charts

- **Contraindications:** Known sensitivity to specific essential oil

* Keep peppermint oil, One of the oils that can be put on the skin. Brings oxygen to an area.

Indications	Oils
Acne	Bergamot, Camphor, Chamomile, Juniper, Lavender, Rosemary, Sandalwood, Tea Tree, Thyme
Allergies/asthma	Chamomile, Moroccan blue, Hyssop, Lavender, Marjoram, Benzoin, Cypress, Eucalyptus, Peppermint, Rosemary
Anxiety/depression (irritability)	Balm Mint/Citrus Oil, Rosemary, Peppermint, Eucalyptus, Rose, Lavender, Chamomile, Moroccan blue, Vetivert, Juniper, Tangerine, Basil, Camphor, Clary sage, Jasmine, Orange blossom, Patchouli, Rose
Arthritis	Benzoin, Birch, Chamomile, Ginger, Juniper, Marjoram, Rosemary
Autoimmune disorders	Vetivert
Blepharitis	Lavender
Boils	Chamomile, Clary sage, Lavender
Bronchitis	Benzoin, Chamomile, Moroccan Blue, Bergamot, Camphor, Eucalyptus, Sandalwood, Frankincense, Lavender, Palmarosa, Tea tree, Peppermint, Rosemary.
Burns	Chamomile, Camphor, Eucalyptus, Lavender, Geranium, Rosemary
Carbuncles	Bergamot, Frankincense, Lavender
Colds	Eucalyptus, Marjoram, Peppermint, Rosemary
Colic	Cardamom, Fennel, Lavender

Colitis	Chamomile
Conjunctivitis	Lavender, Rose
Dermatitis	Chamomile, Moroccan blue, Lavender, Juniper, Peppermint, Cedarwood, Geranium, Jasmine, Rosemary, Rosewood, Sage, Spearmint
Eczema	Juniper, Bergamot, Lavender, Chamomile, Cedarwood, Patchouli, Rose, Rosemary, Sage
Fatigue	Basil, Geranium, Lavender
Fungal infections	Palmarosa, Tea tree, Cedarwood
Hangover	Fennel, Juniper, Rosemary
Hemorrhage	Rose, Immortelle, Cypress, Eucalyptus, Frankincense, Myrrh, Rose
Hemorrhoids	Cypress, Frankincense, Juniper
Herpes	Eucalyptus
Hormonal regulator	Vetivert, Rose, Clary sage, Lavender
Hypertension	Rosemary, Chamomile, Moroccan blue, Lavender, Lemon, Marjoram, Ylang-ylang
Immune System	Lemon, Tea Tree
Impotence/frigidity	Clary sage, Jasmine, Rose, Ylang-ylang, Clove, Ginger, Nutmeg, Pepper, Peppermint, Sandalwood
Inflammation/ infections	Peppermint, Eucalyptus, Chamomile, Moroccan blue, Rose, Lavender, Lemon, Immortelle, Tea tree, Frankincense, Myrrh

Influenza	Camphor, Eucalyptus, Cypress, Peppermint, Rosemary
Insomnia	Chamomile, Lavender, Juniper, Tangerine, Marjoram, Orange blossom, Rose, Sandalwood, Ylang-ylang
Laryngitis	Benzoin, Frankincense, Sandalwood
Lethargy	Lemon, Peppermint, Tea tree, Lavender, Meadow flower, Thyme, Sage
Migraine	Angelica, Basil, Eucalyptus, Lavender, Marjoram, Peppermint, Rosemary, Chamomile, Ginger
Muscle spasms/ cramps	Lavender, Rosemary, Peppermint, Juniper, Basil, Birch, Clove
Neuralgia	Eucalyptus, Peppermint, Bay, Clove
Neuritis, sciatica, fibromyalgia	Chamomile, Moroccan Blue, Juniper
Pain	Rosemary, Peppermint, Chamomile, Moroccan blue, Lavender, Juniper, Bergamot
Psoriasis	Bergamot, Lavender
Perspiration	Clary, Cypress, Lavender, Sage
Respiratory Infections	Bay, Cedarwood, Clove, Cypress, Eucalyptus, Lavender, Peppermint, Pine, Rosemary, Spearmint, Spruce, Tea Tree
Rheumatism	Camphor, Cypress, Eucalyptus, Juniper, Lavender, Rosemary, Birch, Ginger
Scabies	Bergamot, Lavender, Peppermint, Rosemary
Schizoid states	Clary sage, Tea tree

Seborrhea	Bergamot, Patchouli, Sage
Sensitive skin/ Sunburn	Chamomile
Shingles	Peppermint
Sinusitis	Basil, Peppermint, Eucalyptus, Palmarosa, Tea tree
Sprains	Camphor
Sunstroke	Lavender
Thrombosis/ ecchymosis/ atherosclerosis -	Immortelle
Toothache	Clove, Camphor, Peppermint
Ulcers (skin)	Eucalyptus, Juniper, Myrrh
Urinary tract infection	Bergamot, Sandalwood, Cedarwood, Eucalyptus, Fir, Juniper, Pine, Tea Tree
Varicose Veins	Cypress
Wounds (Antiseptic)	Bergamot, Lavender, Eucalyptus, Sandalwood, Basil, Benzoin, Eucalyptus, Frankincense, Juniper, Lavender, Myrrh, Patchouli, Rosemary

**When blending more than one essential oil--keep total number of drops to 8 or 10.

Relaxing /Stress Reduction Aromatherapy Steam Bath

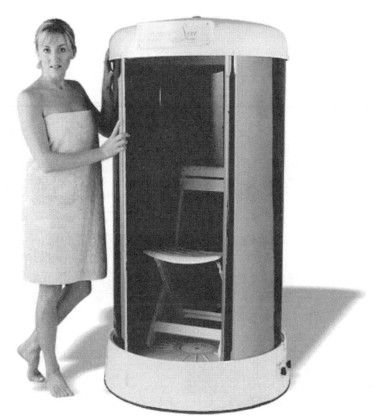

Aroma Spa - Courtesy of Steam Embrace

- Description   Wet or Steam aromatherapy bath using a tub or cabinet.

- Rationale: Sedative, relaxing, calming

- Equipment: Bathtub or Steam cabinet as above with addition of premixed oils or some combination of the following oils added to water: Chamomile - 2 drops; Cypress - 4 drops; Orange blossom - 2 drops; Lavender - 4 drops; Marjoram - 4 drops; Rose - 2 drops; Sandalwood - 4 drops; Clary sage - 4 drops. Balm mint and Valerian are also commonly used in relaxing formulas.

- Procedure: Same as above aromatherapy baths.

- Indications: Insomnia, hyperactivity, anxiety, stress.

- Contraindications: Hypersensitivity to aromatic herbs/oils

148

Tonic / Stimulating Aromatherapy Bath

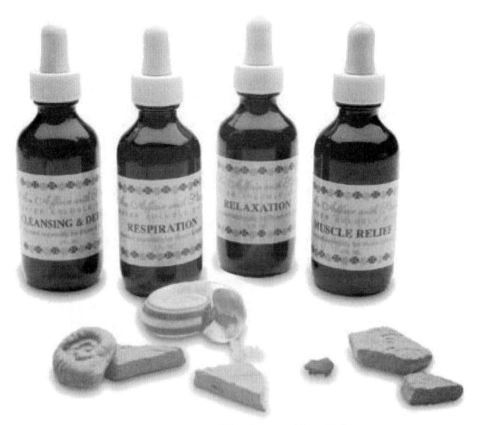

Water Soluble Aromatherapy Oils - Courtesy of Steam Embrace

- **Description:** Wet or Steam aromatherapy bath using a tub or cabinet.

- **Rationale:** Stimulating, invigorating, increases circulation.

- **Equipment:** The same as the above aromatherapy baths with the addition of premixed oils or some combination of the following oils: basil - 3 drops; cardamom - 3 drops; peppermint - 3 drops; juniper - 4 drops; hyssop - 3 drops; rosemary - 4 drops.

- **Procedure:** Same as above.

- **Indications:** Lethargy, depression

- **Contraindications:** Hypersensitivity to Aromatic herbs/oils.

Aromatherapy Facial Steam

- **Description:** Essential oils are added to a facial steaming device.

- **Rationale:** Fragrance and oils can stimulate or sedate circulation and respiratory membranes.

- **Equipment:** Heatproof bowl or commercial steaming device. Essential oils. Towels.

- **Procedure:** Add essential oils, according to skin type, to a bowl containing 1 ½ quarts of boiling water. Breathe deeply and Remain under steam for 10 minutes.

  Normal skin: 2 drops - lavender or geranium;
  Sensitive skin: 2 drops - chamomile or lavender;
  Oily skin: 2 drops - juniper or tea tree;
  Dry skin: 2 drops - sandalwood or patchouli;
  Mature skin: 2 drops - lavender or frankincense.

Modern Facial Steamer

- **Indications:** Above skin conditions.

- **Contraindications:** Hypersensitivity to Aromatic herbs/oils.

Carbon Dioxide Baths

- **Description:** An immersion bath modified by mixing various gases and solid substances with the water. Some are found naturally, such as Saratoga Springs (USA) or created by special mixing apparatus.

- **Rationale:** Circulation is increased by carbon dioxide entering the skin. Circulation to organs decreases, the heart is slowed, and blood pressure normalizes (if high, lowers & if low, raises), respiratory and pulse rates slow down, and elimination of urine increases.

- **Equipment:** Natural springs or perforated tubes are placed in the bottom of the tub and carbon dioxide flows into the water. Production of carbon dioxide water requires 4-8 pounds of salt, 1/2 pound of sodium bicarbonate, and 6-8 large tablets of acid sodium sulfate.

- **Procedure:** Baths are administered daily. Progressively increase the percentage of carbon dioxide, beginning with 25%, then 50%, 75%, and finally 100%.

  Mix the salt with 40 gallons of water in a tub, add the sodium bicarbonate and then place the acid sodium sulfate tablets at equal intervals in the tub.

  The bath temperature begins at 95 F. and subsequent baths are reduced in temperature to no lower than 80 F. The duration of the first bath is 10 minutes and eventually increased up to 15 minutes. The patient lies quietly in the bath.

- **Indications:** Hypertension, advanced cardiac disease, nervous irritability, and insomnia.

- **Contraindications:** Heart disease with decompensation, arteriosclerosis.

Oxygen Bath

- **Description:** Oxygen (or ozone) from a tank or generator is bubbled into the water from perforated tubes lying at the bottom of the tub.

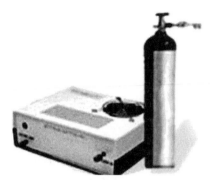

Ozone Generator - Courtesy of Steam Embrace

- **Rationale:** The hyper-oxygenated water may contribute oxygen to superficial tissue and exert a stimulating effect on soft tissues while exerting a soothing effect on the nervous system.

- **Equipment:** Tub, oxygen tank, perforated tubing.

- **Procedure:** The water temperature is held between 91 and 95 F. and full body baths should last from 10-20 minutes.

- **Indications:** Hypertension, advanced cardiac disease, peripheral vascular disease, diabetes, nervous irritability, and insomnia.

- **Contraindications:** Heart disease with decompensation, arteriosclerosis, infectious skin disease.

Brine or Salt Bath

- Description: Artificial brine baths are made by adding sodium chloride to water, causing the patient to be very buoyant.

- Rationale: The buoyancy is soothing and the hypertonic bath solution may cause osmosis of fluids into the skin from deeper tissues.

- Equipment: 5-8 pounds of sodium chloride added to 40 gallons of water **or** artificial seawater can be made by mixing: 7 pounds of sodium chloride, one pound of magnesium chloride, and 1/2 pound of magnesium sulfate in 30 gallons of water in a tub.
Weights may be necessary to hold patient down.

- Procedure: Mix the desired additives to the water.
Water temperature is 90-105 F.
The patient lies in the bath from 10-20 minutes.

- Indications: Osteomyelitis, fractures, dislocations, arthritis, myositis, fibrositis, gout, chronic sciatica, and obesity.

- Contraindications: Arteriosclerosis, cardiac disease, hypertension, and skin rashes or inflammation.

Mint & Sea Salt Bath

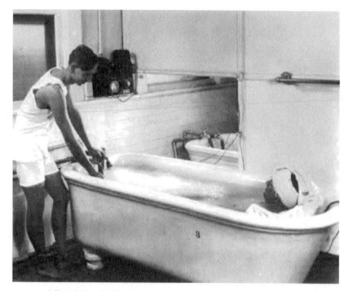

Mint & Sea Salt Bath - Battlecreek Sanitarium - Circa 1925

- **Description:** Mint and Dead Sea salts are used as an additive to the bath to achieve the desired effects.

- **Rationale:** Mineral content and mint are stimulating to the circulation and cleansing to superficial tissue.

- **Equipment:** Tub of warm water.
Additives -- mint and sea salt
Blanket.

- **Procedure:** Mix 2 ounces of the mint sea salt with 4 cups warm water.
Swirl and dissolve in tub of warm (102 degrees F) bath water.
Submerge and bathe for 10-20 minutes.
Rinse with cool/cold shower.
Wrap in warm blanket and rest for 10-20 minutes.

- **Indications:** Dry skin, fatigue.

- **Contraindications:** Hypersensitivity to aromatic herbs/oils.

154

Steam Bath

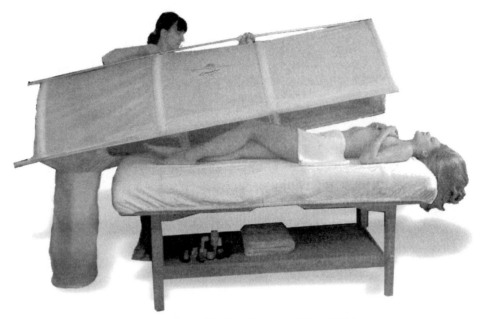

Steamy Wonder - Courtesy of Steam Embrace

- Description: Steam baths are hyperthermic procedures. They are intended for the healthy and thought to be preventive and strengthening. Heat is produced in an enclosed structure. Water can be thrown on heated stones to create steam. There are also manufactured steam tubs. The bath is followed by a cold, drenching bath or dip in a cool pool. After sweating has been induced, the running water or dip in the pool concludes this bath.

- Rationale: In an attempt to increase heat loss through the skin and lungs, sweating increases and reflexive hormonal and nervous system changes occur to increase the heat loss. The metabolic rate increases 12-20%, pulse rate increases 30-40% (less as a person becomes accustomed to these baths). There are changes in arterial blood pressure, an increase of 60% venous blood pressure in healthy subjects, and varying losses of electrolyte content through sweating. Skeletal and smooth muscle, as well as connective tissue, relax in response to heat.

- Equipment: Steam cabinet or canopy (as shown above).

- **Procedure:**   Client sits in steam room for 5-15 minutes.
Temperature is between 128-150 degrees F.
Breathe deeply.
Friction or loofah rub can be added to exfoliate dead skin.
Follow treatment with cool to cold shower (or cold plunge).
Limit treatment to 10-15 minutes because of dehydration.
Drink plenty of fluids before and after treatment.

- **Indications:**   Pain, muscle spasms, bronchial congestion, cleansing of skin and anxiety/agitation.

- **Contraindications:** Heat speeds up the chemical processes in the body. The pulse rate increases from 75 beats per minute to between 100-150 beats per minute during a 15-20 minute treatment. Therefore, increased cardiovascular activities are not recommended for people with heart disease or other cardiovascular problems. People with high blood pressure or diabetes with peripheral vascular disease should consult their physician.

Sauna Bath

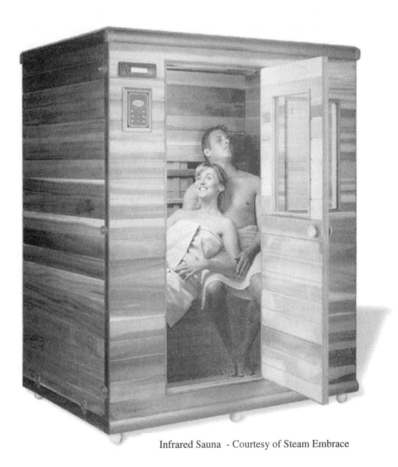

Infrared Sauna - Courtesy of Steam Embrace

- **Description:**   Enclosed structure with a heating device. The air is dry, and this procedure is hyperthermic--also considered preventive and strengthening. The procedures are the same as for the steam bath. Scents can be distributed through the enclosure by an aromatherapy device. Eucalyptus oil is well known for its effect in preventing and relieving catarrhal discomfort. Pine needle scent (contains pine needle and citrus oils) is invigorating and revitalizing. Menthol oil deodorizes and clears sinus passages.

- **Rationale:**   Relaxing, stimulates metabolism and circulation, induces perspiration and cleansing, stimulates immune system and helps prevent upper bronchial infections. Skeletal and smooth muscle, as well as connective tissue, relax with heat.

- Equipment: Sauna unit, either conventional or Far-Infrared.

- Procedures: Air temperature ranges from 60-90 degrees C. The relative humidity is only 5-10%. Humidity is maintained by spraying water mixed with sauna scents over hot stones of the sauna oven. Mix 2 parts of sauna scent to 5 parts of water.

  Cleanse body with warm water (opens pores) before entering.

  The sauna phase usually lasts 10-20 minutes and is followed by a cooling phase. These phases are usually alternated 2-3 times. Begin sitting on the lower benches and gradually move upwards. Between 400-1,000 grams of perspiration is usually lost in a sauna bath. (**Important to rehydrate**.)

  The cooling phase begins by sitting in cool air and then a cool shower and finally a short plunge in a cold pool of water. Include the head in the cooling process to avoid a headache. The cooling phase closes the pores and vessels of the skin.

  Rest with legs elevated for 10-15 minutes. Then re-enter the sauna. This process is repeated 2-3 times.

  Limit treatment to 10-15 minutes because of dehydration. Drink plenty of fluids before and after treatment.

- Indications: Colds, flu, sinusitis or other respiratory problems. Muscle spasm and hypertonicity.

- Contraindications: Heat speeds up the chemical processes in the body. The pulse rate increases from 75 beats per minute to between 100-150 beats per minute during a 15-20 minute treatment. Therefore, increased cardiovascular activities are not recommended for people with heart disease or other cardiovascular problems. People with high blood pressure or diabetes with peripheral vascular disease, should consult their physician.

  * See Far Infrared Sauna and Hyperthermia on page 193.

158

G. Ablutions

> Ablutions are the mildest form of Kneipp water application, performed by pouring or using a wet cloth to cleanse and wash.   Ablutions differ from the usual cleansing procedures because the washing procedure is divided into whole and part body washings. Ablutions are usually divided into: upper extremities, chest and back; lower extremities, buttocks; whole body and abdomen.

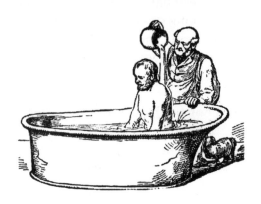

Ablution--Upper extremities, Chest, and Back

- **Description:**   A wet cloth is dampened and used to wash the upper extremities, chest, and back area.

- **Rationale:**   Enhances blood circulation and is relaxing. The body produces heat and the elimination of metabolic waste products in the blood is increased.

- **Equipment:**   Wash cloth.
Dish cold water.
One part vinegar to two parts of water.

- **Procedure:**   Insure that the room is draft-free and warm.
Dip washcloth in cold water and wash as follows:

  1. Right arm - first exterior to the shoulder, the hand, then the interior armpit.

  2. Left arm - the same procedure as right arm.

3. Across the chest, and then a clockwise stroke across the abdomen.

4. The backside (thoracic down to gluteal area) is rubbed down with several strokes.

The procedure is completed as quickly as possible. Do not dry. Instead, redress in warm clothing or wrap in towel and rest for 10-15 minutes (staying warm).

- Indications: Stress syndrome, dysfunction of the thermoregulatory system, rheumatism, colds, insomnia, and fever.

- Contraindications: Oversensitivity to cold.

Ablution--Lower Extremities, Buttocks

- Description: Washing of the lower extremities and buttocks area.

- Rationale: Same as above.

- Equipment: Same as above.

- Procedure: Same as above with the following exceptions:

    The direction of the wash follows these guidelines:

    1. Right leg - first exterior front.

    2. Left leg - front.

    3. Right leg - back.

    4. Left leg - back.

    5. Soles of the feet.

- Indications: Same as above with addition of varicose veins.

- Contraindications: Same as above.

Ablution--Whole Body

- **Description:** Same as above except entire body is washed.

- **Rationale:** Stimulate blood flow/circulation/immune system or quiet/relax nerves.

- **Equipment:** Same as above.

- **Procedure:** Dip washcloth into cold water and wash:

  1. Right arm front - exterior then interior.
  2. Left arm front - exterior then interior.
  3. Throat, across chest, and then clockwise strokes across abdomen.
  4. Right leg - front, start with foot.
  5. Left leg - front, start with foot.
  6. Back side - is washed down with several strokes.
  7. Right leg back - start with the heel.
  8. Left leg back - start with the heel.
  9. Right and left soles of the feet.

  Complete as quickly as possible.
  Wrap in warm blanket or redress & stay warm for 10-20 minutes.

- **Indications:** Bedridden patients, immune deficiency, chronic rheumatic disease, insomnia, poor circulation.

- **Contraindications:** Over sensitivity to cold.

Ablution --Abdomen

- **Description:** Same as above, but only stomach area involved.

- **Rationale:** Stimulates digestive organs.

- **Equipment:** Same as above. Warm bed.

- **Procedure:** Bend patient's knees and keep warm in bed.
  Dip washcloth into cold water.
  Rub abdomen with washcloth clockwise 20-40 times.
  Immerse washcloth several times during treatment.
  Continue treatment for five minutes.

- Indications: Bedridden patients, immune deficiency, chronic rheumatic disease, insomnia, poor circulation.

- Contraindications: Over sensitivity to cold.

H. Affusions

> Affusions are a mild form of Kneipp water application performed by the pouring of water in a stream, or with a hose without using pressure. Affusions are usually divided into: upper extremities, chest and back; lower extremities, buttocks; whole body; and abdomen.

Cold Knee Affusion

- Description: Cold water is applied to the knee area by an unpressurized hose.

- Rationale: Blood pressure is reduced, arterial blood flow increased, and venous blood flow is stimulated.

- Equipment: Hose and water source. Hose is 3/4 inch wide and 3 ½ ft. long. Warm blanket or wrapping.

- Procedure: Water is 65 degrees F.

  Client inhales and exhales evenly during the affusion. Begin distally on the **right** leg, posterior side. Begin at the lateral side of foot. Hose upwards along the calf 3/4 inches above the popliteal space. Hold this position until the skin turns red, then move downward on the **medial** side of the calf to the heel.

  Repeat the same stroke on the **left** leg as described above. Hold the position above the popliteal space until the skin turns red. Then, change the affusion from the left knee cap to the right and back to the left. Proceed down the medial left leg as described above.

  Client continues to inhale and exhale evenly during the affusion. Repeat process on anterior side of lower legs. Begin with the

right leg, **lateral** side and repeat process as described above.
Repeat the same stroke on the **left** leg. Again, stay with the
affusion above the knee and change from the left knee cap to the
right, and back to the left again. Then proceed down the **medial**
side of the left calf to the toes.

Conclude with circular affusion on the bottom of both feet.
Wipe water off with hands (do not towel dry). Follow with
active exercise to keep legs warm or wrap in socks and cover
with warm blanket in bed.

- Indications: Vascular headaches, poor blood circulation in legs, varicose
veins, elevated body temperature.

- Contraindications: Menstruation, sciatic pain, bladder or kidney infection, cold
feet, over-sensitivity to cold, or low blood pressure.

Knee Affusion, Alternate Temperature

- Description: Same as above, but temperature alternates between warm and cold.

- Rationale: Reduces blood pressure, increases arterial blood flow, relaxes
and relieves insomnia.

- Equipment: Same as above, but water temperature must be regulated.

- Procedure:
  1. Warm affusion, Posterior -- 97-100 degrees F.
  Procedure is the same as above, except the affusion is held
  above the knee until the client feels warm and a light redness
  appears. The process as described above is repeated on the right
  and then the left leg.

  2. Warm affusion, Anterior -- 97-100 degrees F.
  Procedure is the same as above, except the affusion is held
  above the knee until the client feels warm and a light redness
  appears. The process as described above is repeated on the
  right and then the left leg.

  3. Cold affusion, Posterior -- 65 degrees F.
  Procedure same as described in cold knee affusion.

  4. Cold affusion, Anterior -- 65 degrees F.
  Procedure same as described in cold knee affusion.

  5. Repeat the warm affusion.

6. Repeat the cold affusion.

7. Finish with cold circular affusion on the bottom of both feet.

8. Wipe off water. Do not towel dry. Wrap the body and keep it warm. Rest for one hour

- Indications: Vascular headaches, poor blood circulation in the legs, elevated body temperature, chronic cold feet.

- Contraindications: Menstruation, sciatic pain, bladder or kidney infection, varicose veins, low blood pressure, or persistent chills.

Leg Affusion , Cold Temperature

- Description: Cold water stream directed at legs in particular direction.

- Rationale: Reduces blood pressure, increases arterial blood flow, stimulates venous blood flow, and relaxes.

- Equipment: ¾ inch hose, 3 ½ feet long.
Water supply.
Blanket.
Water temperature 65 degrees F.

- Procedure: The client inhales and exhales evenly throughout the affusion. Begin on the right lateral side of the **posterior right** foot. Hose upwards along the lateral side of the leg to the gluteal area. Maintain position until the skin reddens, then move downwards along the medial side of the leg to the heel. Repeat the same stroke on the left leg. Stay with the affusion on the gluteals and change from the left side to the right, and then back to the left side. Continue hosing downward along the medial left leg to the heel.

  The affusion is then completed as described above on the anterior legs. The procedure begins on the lateral side of the **right** foot and moves superiorly to the inguinal ligament. Maintain this position until the skin appears red. Move downward along the medial side of the leg to the toes. Repeat this same stroke on the left leg. Stay with the affusion on the inguinal ligament space, changing from the left side to the right, and then back to the left. Continue hosing downward on the medial side of the left leg to the toes.

Conclude with cold circular affusion on the bottom of both feet. Wipe water off by hand. Follow the affusion with exercise or one hour of bed rest, keeping the client warm.

- Indications: Unstable cardiovascular system, varicose veins, poor blood circulation in the legs.

- Contraindications: Menstruation, oversensitivity to cold, sciatic pain, bladder/kidney infection, cold feet, low blood pressure.

Leg Affusion, Alternate Temperature

- Description: Stream of water applied to legs, alternating temperature.

- Rationale: Reduces blood pressure, enhances blood circulation, increases arterial blood flow, stimulates venous blood flow, and relaxes.

- Equipment: Same as above.

- Procedure: Applied in the same fashion as described above. Begin with a warm affusion (97-100 degrees F), applying it to the posterior side and then the anterior side as described above. Apply a cold affusion (65 degrees F) to the posterior and then anterior side as described above.

  Repeat the warm and then the cold affusion.

  Conclude in same manner as previously described.

- Indications: Poor blood circulation, insomnia.

- Contraindications: Menstruation, sciatic pain, bladder/kidney infection, and over-sensitivity to cold.

I. Showers

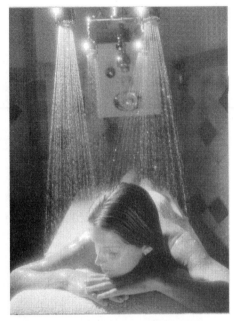

Modern Vichy Shower - Courtesy of Hydro Spa Consulting

A shower is defined as an application of water by an apparatus that drives or throws water on the surface of the body at different striking pressures and temperatures.
Various types of showers are described below:

Jet Shower

- **Description:** Therapeutic shower using multiple high pressure nozzles and varied water temperatures.

- **Rationale:** To stimulate by increasing blood circulation to an area.

- **Equipment:** Specially designed shower device or garden hose with nozzle and water supply. Towels.

- **Procedures:** The operator holds hose and stands 9 feet from the patient. The water is directed between the shoulder blades, up and down the back, and finally up and down the extremities. The water temperature may be neutral to begin with, and can be adjusted up or down depending on the desired outcome. The pressure can be raised or lowered depending on the amount of stimulation desired (similar to Scotch Shower).

- **Indications:** Conditions of reduced vitality and poor circulation. Often used after a heat treatment or massage.

- **Contraindications:** Chilled Patient

Fan Shower

- **Description:** Therapeutic shower using multiple nozzles arranged in a fan shaped array and varied water temperatures.

- **Rationale:** To stimulate by increasing blood circulation to an area.

- **Equipment:** Same as above, but with a fan device on hose, or the operator can use their finger to "fan" the water. The jet and fan shower can be alternated, depending on the desired affect.

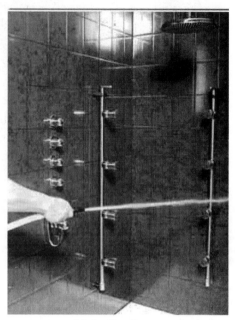

Modern Fan Shower

- **Procedures:** The operator holds hose and stands 9 feet from the patient. The water is directed between the shoulder blades, up and down the back, and finally up and down the extremities. The water temperature may be neutral to begin and can be adjusted up or down depending on the desired outcome. The pressure can be raised or lowered depending on the amount of stimulation desired (Similar to Scotch Shower).

- **Indications:** Conditions of reduced vitality and poor circulation. Often used after a heat treatment or massage.

- **Contraindications:** Chilled Patient

Rain Shower

- **Description:** Same as above with water pipes are arranged with many outlets in a circular, triangular or quadrilateral manner. The pipes contain varied temperatures of water as well as different intensities. The arrangement allows for water to be thrown against the body at many different levels, with different temperatures and intensities (also called the horizontal rain or needle shower).

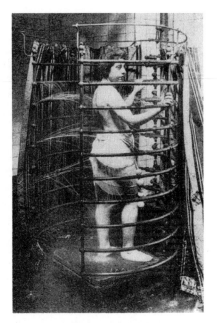

Rain Shower - Circa 1920

- **Rationale:** To stimulate by increasing blood circulation to an area.

- **Equipment:** Specially designed shower device or garden hose, with multiple nozzle and water supply. Towels.

- **Procedures:** Patient stands in shower for 5-10 minutes, depending on desired effects.

- **Indications:** Conditions of reduced vitality and poor circulation. Often used after a heat treatment or massage.

- **Contraindications:** Chilled Patient

Scotch Shower / Blitz Guss

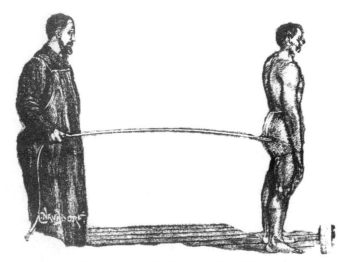

Scotch or Percussion Shower - Circa 1900

- **Description:** Treatment also known as a Scotch Douche, Percussion Douche, or Percussion Shower. Involves the application of a pressurized stream or column of water directed against a portion of the body in a specific sequence.

- **Rationale:** This shower increases mental alertness and has a "tonic" affect, due to the pressure and duration of the water striking the body.

- **Equipment:** Same as for sprays with the addition of a percussion nozzle and controls.

- **Procedures:** The operator stands approximately 9 feet from the patient. The water pressure and temperature are varied. Usually hot water is applied for 1-3 minutes, followed by cold (usually 1/4 the time as the hot application). The hot water ranges from 38 to 50 C. and the cold from 13 to 22 C. The shower begins with hot water at 38 C. applied for one minute, followed by cold water at 27 C. applied for ten seconds. Each day the hot water can be made a degree hotter until 40 C. is reached. The cold is lowered 1.5 C. each day until 11 C. is reached. The patient's response can guide the duration and rate of change of temperature.

  The sequence and pattern of body parts sprayed is as follows:

Application Sequence for Scotch or Percussion Shower

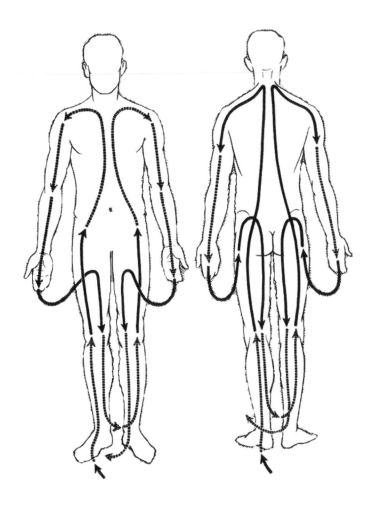

**Dashed lines represent Fanning Spray and
Solid lines represent Jet Spray**

- Indications: Conditions of reduced vitality and poor circulation. Often used after a heat treatment or massage.

- Contraindications: Chilled Patient.

Vichy Shower

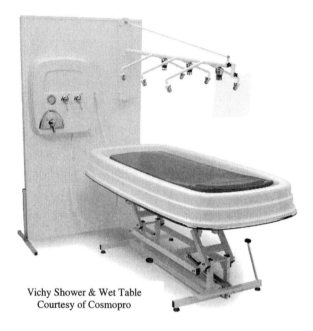

Vichy Shower & Wet Table
Courtesy of Cosmopro

- Description: Similar to Rain Shower with shower device over the patient.

- Rationale: Stimulating or relaxing, depending on pressure and temperature of the water applied. Acts by increasing circulation and nervous activity, relaxation of muscle, and connective tissue.

- Equipment: Wet Table, Vichy, or Spray apparatus.

- Procedure: The patient lies on the Wet Table.

   Tonic: A fan spray is applied to the sides of the trunk and abdomen (avoid gall bladder area) at a temperature of 36 C. in the beginning, and raising the temperature to 41 C. in 3-5 minutes. The patient then stands, and a short, partial jet spray shower is applied.

   Sedative: Water is applied to the abdomen at 36 to 37 C. with almost no pressure for 2-4 minutes in a circular or spiral motion. Normally, the patient then stands and a short, partial jet spray shower is applied.

- Indications: Conditions of reduced vitality and poor circulation. Often used after a heat treatment, massage, or mud/seaweed wrap.

- Contraindications: Chilled Patient

J. Wraps

Paraffin Hydrating Body Wrap

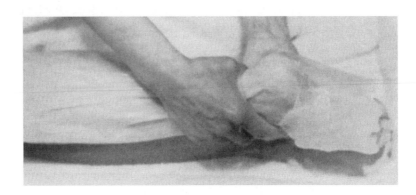

- **Description:**   A paraffin mixture is applied to the body, first the anterior
  side and then the posterior side. The application is
  preceded by an exfoliating dry brush rub and massage.
  It can be customized with various essential oils and scented
  paraffin. The paraffin effectively heats the tissue and muscles.

- **Rationale:**   Stimulating and relaxing, analgesic

- **Equipment:**   Japanese body brush or Loofah mitt
  Massage table
  Paraffin bath (120 - 130 degrees F)
  Candy thermometer
  7-8 bath towels (one to cover treatment table)
  12"x 24" precut tissues (18-20)
  Blanket
  Moisturizing spray
  Massage oil as well as essential oils
  Body powder

  **Paraffin is extremely flammable and should only be heated in
  a UL-listed unit built specifically for this purpose.

  Pure paraffin is completely harmless to the skin. However,
  scented waxes are available (peach and wintergreen are very
  popular). Make sure your client has no any skin
  sensitivities if using anything other than pure paraffin.

- **Procedure:**   Check paraffin for proper temperature and cover massage
  table with bath towel. Have client lie prone on massage table

with proper draping. Check with client for areas of **special** consideration. Additional layers of paraffin can be added to those areas.

Mist the body area being treated before dry brushing the area. All brushing is done with **upward** strokes. Begin with the right side of the body and move toward the heart. Starting with the bottom of the feet, brush the client's feet, legs, thighs and back. Work from the waist up to the shoulders and out to the arms. If any **redness** develops, **stop**. Be aware of the client's preferences and skin type. The length of time should be adjusted accordingly. The legs are usually brushed from one to five minutes. The same is true for the upper back and arm areas.

Essentials oils are mixed with massage oil. Normally one ounce of basic massage oil is mixed with 1-8 drops of each essential oil. Massage with light effleurage movements. The massage lasts 5-10 minutes and follows the same patterns described for dry brushing.

Dip pre-cut tissues into paraffin. Let excess paraffin drip off and apply to body. *Be cautious of temperature--if too hot, let cool a few seconds before applying. Begin with right leg (including the heel) and wrap the leg from heel to thigh. Then cover the leg with a bath towel. Do the same for the left leg. Apply and mold paraffin-coated tissues to the back, shoulders, neck and upper arms down to the elbow. Cover with a towel and then with a blanket. The client then rests for 10 minutes. The blanket, towels, and paraffin tissues are removed from the body. Roll up the paraffin tissues, beginning with the feet, and proceed up the body.

The client then turns over and is supine, with proper draping. Repeat the misting of the body, dry brushing, and massage as described in the above steps. Begin with the toes of the right foot and move up the leg to the thighs. Repeat with the left leg. Lightly brush the stomach and chest area. Brush the fingertips and arms toward the shoulders. Do not brush the palms of the hands.

Massage the body areas treated. Beginning with the right leg, prepare and apply paraffin-dipped tissues as described above. Follow the same order as described in Step 11. Be sure to cover the ankles, knees, and sides of the hip. Cover with a towel. Then proceed to the stomach and chest area. Beginning with the right arm, wrap the entire arm, including the hands and finger. Cover the client with a blanket. The client rests for 10 minutes.

Remove the blanket and towels. Beginning with the right leg and moving upward, roll up paraffin tissues. Powder the client's feet **before standing** to prevent slipping.

- Indications: Low back pain, menstrual pain, colds and congestion, dry skin, arthritis, bursitis, tendonitis, over-worked and fatigued muscles, eczema, and psoriasis.

- Contraindications: Sensitive skin, a rash, claustrophobia, heart problems, and high blood pressure.

Mud and Seaweed Wraps, Scrubs and Polishes

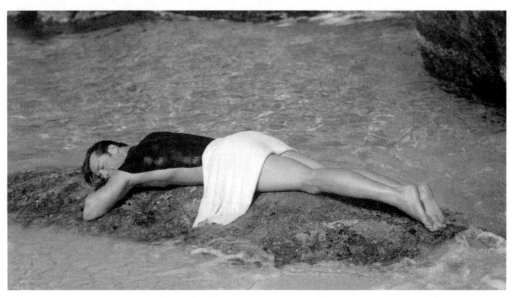

Peloid/Mud Wrap - Courtesy of Pevonia

- Description: Peloids (from a word meaning resembles mud) are found in lakes, moors, rivers, and on the ocean floor. The terms peat, mud, and earth all refer to peloids. According to the German Spa Association, muds are divided into four categories--bath peats, fangos, biogenous sediments, and healing earths. Peat consists of decomposed vegetable parts and are dark brown and rich in carbon; fangos are silts and bluish-gray in color and the minerals correspond to the composition of the water. Fangocean contains ocean floor silt composed of both organic (plant) and inorganic (life) materials, which contain all the minerals of the ocean. Biogenous sediment are found in mineral springs, which contains the minerals of the spring, earth, and bacteria.

  Seaweeds are marine algae and classified by color--browns, greens, reds, blue-greens, yellow-greens and white. Seaweed contains all the minerals required by man and more than any other plant food--from 7 to 33% of their dry weight. Browns are predominately antibacterial, cleansing, and regenerative; greens are used for their firming qualities; whites re-mineralize and relax; reds are hydrating and nourishing, and are used as vermicides.

  The various "menus" for wraps, packs, scrubs, and polishes depend on the client's individual needs. Body scrubs are stimulating and remove dead skin cells; body polishes soften, refine, and re-mineralize the skin; seaweed body wraps are relaxing, rejuvenating, and in some cases designed for specific problems; mud wraps are designed to balance the skin, promote relaxation and a sense of well-being, and hormonal balance. These special treatments require a thorough understanding of the products used and the client's needs. Reputable manufacturers should be used who can guarantee organically pure products, support materials, and "hot-lines" for questions.

- **Rational:** Minerals are necessary for the acid/alkaline balance of the body and skin. Some 32 elements occur in seawater such as calcium, potassium, silicon, magnesium, sulfur, sodium, chlorine, and bromine. These minerals are predominantly revitalizing, hydrating, and relaxing. Each of these muds and seaweeds have its own unique mineral composition and action when used in packs or wraps (as well as baths).

- **Equipment:** Spa table (massage, facial, or wet table).
  Colored shower curtains.
  Natural boar bristle brushes, loofah mitts, bath sponges.
  Wet pillow, knee bolster, headrest.
  Washable blankets.
  Mixing bowls, measuring cups, measuring spoons.
  Astrowrap/spa foil, plastic wrap, cotton sheets.

  Products--powdered or liquid algaes, moor/muds, bath solutions such as algae, moor, essential oils, herbal foams, sea salts and exfoliants such as oatmeal, almond paste, dry brushes, algae gels, and finishing lotions (marine, herbal). The mixture and choice of products used depends on the client's needs.

- Procedure:
    1. Cover table with blanket(s), Astrowrap (spa foil, or plastic) and heated cotton or flannel sheet (may be dipped in herbal solution).
    2. Have client use steam or sauna for 10-20 minutes, then quickly dry brush or scrub with exfoliant mixture.
    3. Apply a thin layer of algae, mud or wrap mixture (per product instructions) to entire body.
    4. Wrap with heated sheet, Astrowrap or plastic, and blanket(s).
    5. Allow client to relax in wrap for 20 - 45 minutes. Remain with client if possible and offer water to drink as needed.
    6. Have client shower with cool water and dry with towel. Apply finishing lotion and allow client to rest for 20 minutes following treatment.

- Indications: See following chart:

Indications	Type of Peloid Used
Hormonal problems detoxify the liver	Peats
Cleanse skin, acne, nutrients for skin, and stimulates the lymphatic system	Fangoceans
Edema, hypertension, gynecological diseases	Brown Seaweed
Toning, hemorrhoids	Green Seaweed
Iodine sensitivity	White Seaweed
Dry skin, respiratory ailments	Red Seaweed

- Contraindications: Skin Sensitivities.

K. Masks

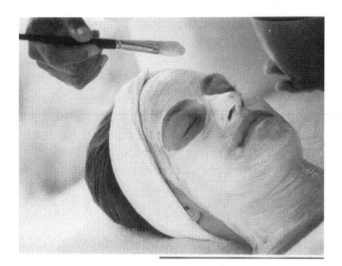

A mask or masque is defined as a skin treatment where the application of mud, seaweed, herbs, paraffin, fruit, etc. are left on the skin for an extended period of time to cleanse, dry, moisturize, exfoliate, or soothe. Various types of masks are described below:

Purifying Body Mask

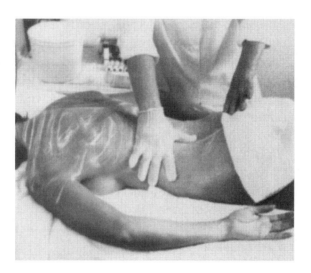

- Description: Application of body scrub to exfoliate dead skin followed by a clay mask which cleanses, firms, tones, and hydrates the skin.

- Rationale: The scrub is stimulating and exfoliating, increasing superficial circulation, and removing superficial cells from the epidermis. The clay application acts by virtue of its hypertonic nature to attract body fluids to the local area and adhere to sweat, oils, or waste products present on the skin surface.

- Equipment: Treatment table
  Egg crate pad
  Electric table warmer
  Dry brush (electric brushing machine optional)
  Shower (optional)
  Body massager (optional)
  Warm water, large washcloths, bath-sized towels, cotton sheets, plastic sheet, 2 small pillows, large hand towels, plastic toweling cut into 3-ft. squares, hair net, exfoliating glove, soft brush, large bowl, large brush, blanket, large bath sponge.
  Mild body scrub and sea clay product. Clay is a blend of Baltic Sea green clay, white English clay, sea minerals, and soothing botanicals.

- Procedure: Place "egg crate" pad on treatment table, followed by electric table warmer. Place cotton sheet followed by plastic sheet on table. Place 4 bath-sized towels over plastic. Towels should hang over side of treatment table. Place small pillow, covered with towel, at head of table. Client lies supine with proper draping. Hair is protected with net.

  Dampen washcloth with warm water and moisten area being treated. Therapist wears exfoliating glove (or soft brush or electric brushing machine). Apply one tablespoon of exfoliating scrub to glove. Begin with arms, then chest area and finally the legs. Upward motions are used. Add more scrub as necessary. Special attention is paid to areas where skin is tough--knees, heels & elbows. Add moisture as needed, as well as changing the warm water when it becomes cloudy.

  Remove the product with large moistened washcloths. Dry each area as you finish the treatment. Fold the towels placed on the table over the arms. Cover the chest area while completing legs to prevent client from becoming chilled. Help client turn over and lie prone. Complete the above treatment on posterior side, beginning with back and ending with legs.

  Mix 1 to 1 1/2 cups of mask into large bowl. While prone, apply sea clay product to back. Beginning with lower back, apply mask with large brush (4"). Upward strokes are used, working toward the shoulders. The application should be thick enough so you are not able to see skin through the mask. Cover the back with pre-cut plastic toweling pieces and form plastic to back. Then begin with the ankles and apply mask to back of the legs up to the hips. Cover with plastic toweling and mold to the body.

Help client turn over on her back, removing the bath towels as she turns, and draping properly. The client will be lying on her back on top of the large plastic sheet. Place a pillow under her knees. Cover client's legs with sheet while applying the mask to the upper body.

Repeat mask application as described above, beginning with the chest, then arms beginning at the wrists and moving to the shoulders--always using upward strokes. Do not apply clay to fingertips as it is difficult to remove. When one side of the body is completed cover with precut plastic toweling and mold to skin. Then apply to stomach area quickly (because it will feel very cool) and cover with plastic toweling molding to body. Cover upper body with sheet and proceed with legs. Peel back the plastic toweling molded to the back of the client's legs. Apply the mask to the legs, beginning at the feet and work toward the hips. Cover this area with plastic toweling.

Remove the cotton sheet from the upper torso. Now wrap the client with the plastic sheet covering the table, creating a cocoon effect. The client will feel the warming effects. Cover with a blanket, dim lights and client rests for 30 minutes.

Remove blanket and plastic sheet. Discard plastic toweling and plastic sheet. If a shower is available, have client use a large bath sponge and remove the product in a warm shower (no soap). If no sponge is available, use clean washcloth dampened with warm water to remove product. Dry with clean towel. Provide a robe and chair while massage table is being cleaned and prepared for massage. Conclude this treatment with a stimulating 3-5 minute massage with either an electric massager or brisk, stimulating massage strokes. The client lies prone. The anterior body is not massaged. Begin the massage with the lower back, moving to the shoulders, then back down to the buttocks, and finally the legs. Finish with the feet. Spend only 30 seconds on any area to avoid over- stimulating.

- Indications: Dry skin, eczema and psoriasis, arthritis, bursitis, tendonitis, over-worked and fatigued muscles.

- Contraindications: Claustrophobia, heart problems, high blood pressure, skin rashes, certain medications (always check with Dr. if client is on any type of medication).

180

Mask Formulas

- Egg Yolk & Honey Facial Mask (best for dry skin types)

  Mix thoroughly: 1 tablespoon Honey
  1 egg yolk
  1/2 teaspoon almond oil
  1 tablespoon plain yogurt
  Allow to penetrate for at least 15 minutes
  Rinse thoroughly with cool water

- Egg Yolk, Avocado & Mud Facial Mask (best for oily skin types)

  Mix thoroughly: 1 tablespoon dry clay, mud or fullers earth
  1 egg yolk
  1/4 mashed avocado
  Witch Hazel sufficient to create a smooth mixture
  Allow to penetrate for at least 15 minutes
  Rinse thoroughly with cool water

- Egg & Olive Oil Hair Mask (best for dry hair)

  Mix thoroughly: 2 whole eggs
  4 tablespoons olive oil
  Smooth through hair and cover with plastic wrap
  Allow to penetrate for at least 10 minutes
  Rinse thoroughly

- Fruit Smoothie Hair Mask (conditioning)

  Blend thoroughly: 1/2 banana
  1/4 avocado
  1/4 cantaloupe
  1 tablespoon wheat germ oil
  1 tablespoon plain yogurt
  Contents of 1 vitamin E capsule
  Smooth through hair and cover with plastic wrap
  Allow to penetrate for at least 15 minutes
  Rinse thoroughly

X. BASIC GUIDELINES

We have discussed the physiological changes that occur from the application of heat and cold, the differences between the two modalities, the expected results, and several factors, which contribute to the results of the treatment. In order to manipulate all the variables, which can be controlled in hydrotherapy, certain factors must be considered in individualizing an effective treatment. The variables that **can be controlled** are:

Temperature: The intensity of the treatment is enhanced by the higher degree of difference between the temperature of the application and the body temperature. For example, the intensity of the treatment increases as the difference in body temperature and application temperatures increase.

Duration: If the temperature of the application is **extreme**, the duration is inversely proportional to the overall intensity of the treatment. For example, very hot or very cold applications are shorter in length of application. Short hot/cold applications stimulate the circulation. Long applications of hot/cold are depressive. A five minute sitz bath at 50 degrees F is more stimulating than a 10 minute sitz bath at 50 degrees F. In contrast, the intensity of a neutral bath (moderate temperature) is increased by the duration of the bath.

Frequency: The intensity of the treatments should increase with the frequency of the applications. Each subsequent treatment's effectiveness is reduced because the body's reactive capacities are reduced with each application.

Timing: The time of the day is important. The treatment is enhanced if given during the patient's strong time. If given during the weak time, the effectiveness is diminished.

Location/Site of Application: The reflex areas discussed are important. Including both the location and the extent of the surface area involved, are important. In a derivative measure, the larger the treatment area, the greater the intensity. In retrostasis, the opposite is true. The smaller the area, the greater the intensity. In contrast therapy, the greater the size of the location treated, the greater the intensity of the treatment.

Pressure vs. Friction:	Pressure is used for affusion or external douche. The greater the force, the greater the intensity of the treatment. The pressure increases the intensity and also increases the patient's tolerance of extreme temperatures.

During an ablution, a strong friction at 45 degrees F is tolerated and more effective than a soft friction at the same temperature. Also, a heavy friction will feel warmer than a light friction.

The pressure and friction compete with, and diminish, the perception of cold. They also bring blood to the surface, which warms cutaneous tissue and quiets cold receptors. |
| **Materials:** | The ability of the water to penetrate the material used in the covering is inversely proportional to the heating effects. Covering a wool compress with plastic cuts down the ability of cooling through evaporation, producing a stronger heating effect and derivative response. |
| **Wetness:** | The wetter the application, the stronger the impact of the temperature on the body. |

To achieve optimum results from each treatment,
several basic rules should be followed. They are:

No surprises: Explain the procedures ahead of time. This explanation includes the length, sequence, frequency, cost, rationale, temperature, etc. Answer your patient's questions.

Take patient's temperature. Adjust the treatment according to the patient's temperature.

Monitor the patient's pulse and temperature during prolonged heat treatments. A strong patient's limits should be less than 140 beats/minute and the temperature below 104 degrees F. A weaker patient would be less.

Chilling - Stop the treatment and warm the patient if he is chilled or shows goose flesh.

Timing - Treat the patient before meals, not immediately after. Also treat the patient during his/her **"strong"** time of the day.

Rest after treatments is very important.

Avoid excess heat after a treatment.

Hot precedes cold (general rule) in a contrast treatment.

Heat applications should cover a **larger** area and **last longer** than cold.

End with cold.

Compress - Cover with wool material.

Contraindications of each treatment must be known. Also consider the patient's health, age, and physical condition. The very young, old, weak, and obese patients require special care, especially during cold applications.

Written records should be clear and kept for prescribed hydrotherapy treatments. It is important to have accurate records for legal reasons, as well as noting what works and what doesn't work. These records are important to insure that the patient receives the very best treatment possible.

XI. FEVER

A. Introduction

A brief discussion of fever is central to understanding hydrotherapy. Fever is defined as an increase in regulated body temperature resulting from an elevation in the thermoregulatory "set point." It is different from elevations in body temperature resulting from exercise, passive heating or heat stroke situations.

Body temperature varies depending on the part of the body where the temperature is taken (rectal temperature is nearly a degree higher than oral temperatures), on the time of day (lowest in morning and highest in late afternoon), on the sex (women's normal temperature is usually higher than men's), and on the state of activity (resting versus after physical exercise).

Hippocrates, the Father of Medicine, said, "Give me fever, and I can cure any disease" because he knew fever stimulated the body's defense system. History documents the beneficial effects of hyperthermia in the form of hot packs, baths, and saunas since 500 B.C. Historically, the intentional injection of a foreign substance, sometimes including the malaria pathogen, was used to create hyperthermia in patients suffering from syphilis and other diseases. Research is currently being conducted into the production of fever by various methods (injection of foreign substances, hot packs, hot baths) in the treatment of health problems ranging from the common cold, to AIDS and cancer.

B. Inducing Hyperthermia by External Applications of Heat

Hyperthermia can be induced by the external application of heat. High-tech approaches use radiant heating via Far Infrared, short-wave or microwave diathermy, ultrasound, and extracorporeal heating.

- **Diathermy** is the application of radio frequency electromagnetic energy to the body causing a rise in the temperature. It is used in localized conditions for treatment of specific tissues.
- **Ultrasound** is the application of high-energy sound waves causing an increase in body temperature, resulting from the friction produced at the molecular level when the sound waves strike body tissues.
- **Radiant Heating** devices produce infrared heat that is applied to the body.
- **Extracorporeal** heating involves removing blood from the body, heating it, and returning it to the body at a higher temperature.

Hyperthermia can be produced locally to treat small areas of infection, or to the entire body to treat a general infection. Whole-body hyperthermia utilizes full-immersion baths, saunas, steam and blanket packs. Hot baths are the simplest method of inducing fever at home as part of a self-care routine. It can be beneficial in treating upper and lower respiratory tract infections. To treat viral infections, hot baths can be combined with hot drinks and blanket-wrapping to stimulate the immune system. A cold wet sheet pack can also be used to produce a therapeutic fever.

Some precautions should be taken. A knowledgeable physician should be consulted prior to undertaking hyperthermia therapy. **Risks of hyperthermia include febrile seizures, spontaneous abortion, radical blood pressure changes, nervous system injury, and acute onset of herpes zoster.** In treating the elderly or very young, extra caution should be used. Patients with the following conditions are also at particular risk: epilepsy, tuberculosis, diabetes, heart disease, peripheral vascular disease, peripheral neuropathy, temperature regulation problems, and pregnancy.

C. Physiological Changes Resulting from Hyperthermia

Fever is a condition due to a disturbance of the heat-regulating mechanism. The usual symptoms of fever are a rise of temperature, increased pulse and breathing rate, and headache. The body is actually treating itself by creating a fever in response to bacterial or viral disease, abnormalities in the brain itself, toxic substances affecting the temperature regulating centers, brain tumors, or dehydration. Many proteins, the by-products of the breakdown of proteins and certain substances secreted by the bacteria (known as pyrogens) can cause the hypothalamic thermostat to rise above the "set point." When this process occurs, all the mechanisms for raising the body temperature are brought into play, including heat conservation and increased heat production.

When the hypothalamic thermostat is suddenly raised, and the blood temperature is less than this new setting, an autonomic response occurs. During this period of time, a person experiences chills, coldness of the skin because of vasoconstriction, and shaking due to shivering. These changes are all an attempt to raise the body temperature. When the blood temperature reaches the same level as the hypothalamic temperature, chills subside. When the hypothalamic thermostat is lowered, the blood temperature is still higher. At this point, vasodilatation occurs, resulting in intense sweating. The skin is hot. The body is attempting to release heat, bringing the blood temperature back in line with the hypothalamic thermostat.

During the phagocytic process, interleukin-l (an endogenous pyrogen) is released. This fever producer travels in the blood to the hypothalamus. The hypothalamus produces prostaglandins that cause the body thermostat to be turned up. Now the body thinks the normal temperature is too low and begins to generate more heat. The body may shiver and begins to conserve heat by vasoconstriction, limiting the blood flow to the cooling surfaces; piloerection shuts down the sweating process. The interleukin-l also causes sleep which helps conserve heat. The liver produces special proteins to aid the immunity. Interleukin-l also goes to skeletal muscle and the prostaglandins are released in the tissue. This is why we "ache" with fever. The muscle tissue breaks down, and the resulting amino acids provide materials for defense, repair, and energy. Interleukin-l also produces a decrease in appetite by decreasing the motility of the organs involved. All these reactions are necessary for the body to survive.

Fever stimulates the immune system. During the fever, circulating white blood cells increase in number. The production, as well as the motility of the WBC's, increases. The production of interferon is increased, also increasing antibody production.

The fever creates a negative environment for the invading organism. Iron and zinc concentration in the blood is reduced, which inhibits bacterial growth. Tissue temperatures of 104 to 106 degrees kill several types of bacteria. A temperature greater than 110 degrees F can result in cell death, depending on the length of time.

D. Fever Management

Fevers usually pass through three stages. During the first stage the patient usually experiences a chill--this feeling of cold may be accompanied by shivering. The skin is cold and pale; the patient may have a headache and experience loss of appetite. The second stage begins about half an hour after the onset of chilling. The skin becomes hot and flushed, and the temperature soon reaches its highest point. Usually after about two to three hours, the patient enters the third stage where the temperature begins to fall. At this time the patient will perspire profusely, urination increases, and the patient begins to feel better.

The temperature fluctuates during a fever. Temperature may drop slowly to normal, a process called lysis (as in typhoid fever). It may drop rapidly to normal, a process called crisis (as in pneumonia). A continued fever is defined as a temperature remaining above normal for several days with little fluctuation. If the temperature remains above normal and fluctuates often, it is called a remittent fever. If the temperature drops to normal at certain times during the day but rises to well above normal at other times, it is called a intermittent fever.

If properly managed, fever will not go to dangerously high levels. Research also shows that fevers rarely go above 104 degrees F in an adult and 105 degrees F in infants and younger children. Antipyretic drugs, such as aspirin, interfere with the fever process. Reye's syndrome in flu and chicken pox has been linked to aspirin use. **A tepid friction rub is the conservative treatment of choice to bring down a fever**. For years mainstream medical thought has dictated that fevers should be reduced immediately with the use of antipyretic drugs. Only in recent years has this issue been openly discussed and options considered.

There can be negative effects of fever. For example, the body's digestive system is shut down. If food is eaten, it strains the digestive system, is not properly digested and uses vital energy needed for defense. Dehydration occurs, as well as electrolyte imbalances, which results in dry skin, dry mouth, and constipation. Research has failed to show any brain damage from fevers, except in the case of meningitis and encephalitis which cause brain damage. Seizures related to fevers are usually the result of the imbalance in electrolytes and dehydration from diarrhea, vomiting, and increased perspiration and respiration. Cold applied to the spine and hot to the head followed by hot to the spine and cold to the head may be helpful in reducing these seizures.

E. Goal of Hydrotherapy in Fever Therapy

The goal of hydrotherapy in treating a fever is to help the body maintain its temperature at the optimal level (generally 102-103 degrees F) while fighting infections. It may be necessary to lower a very high fever, or increase a low fever, facilitating an increase in immunity and improved circulation. Fever therapy is effective in relieving the symptoms of such diseases as arthritis and some skin and neurological disorders. Generally the patient should rest and fast, insuring they receive proper hydration.

Therapists must consider heat production and heat elimination. A short, cold application increases heat loss and heat production, with no appreciable loss in body temperature. A cold, long treatment leads to heat loss combined with a decrease in heat production, and a small loss in body temperature. The heat loss is not as great as you might think because the cold drives the heat-carrying blood to the interior. A tepid application actually results in a larger net heat loss. It is effective because the circulation to the periphery is relatively undisturbed. A long, hot application results in decreased heat elimination and increased heat production. However, a very short hot application of less than a minute increases heat elimination because of vasodilation and perspiration, and result in an insignificant rise in heat production for a small net loss of body heat. The only applications resulting in a net loss of body heat are the long cold, tepid, and very short hot, but the loss is small.

Friction can change the outcome of these treatments. Friction allows the patient to tolerate a cold treatment better and also draws the heat-carrying blood to the skin for increased heat elimination. The blood flow to the muscles and organs is reduced, slowing heat production and the nerves are warmed, cutting down on the reflex production of heat via shivering. Heat is in the blood, not the skin. Friction draws blood to the surface to be cooled. Therefore, cold is not conducive to fever reduction without friction. Also, if the patient begins to shiver, stop your treatment. Shivering increases heat production, decreases heat elimination and raises the temperature you are trying to reduce.

Proper hydration of the patient is very important. Have the patient drink as much as they want unless otherwise indicated. If perspiration is present, external water applications are not necessary. This is the body's mechanism for reducing fever.

Tepid affusion (81-92 degrees F) or neutral affusion (93-96 degrees F), tepid or neutral bath, graduated bath, Brand bath, hot evaporating sheet, and tepid sponge bath are common treatments used in fever reduction.

F. Summary of Fever Producing & Reducing Techniques

The following chart compares the temperature of the application, the duration of the application, heat elimination, heat production, and any net change in body temperature.

Temperature / Length of Application	Heat Elimination	Heat Production	Net Temperature Change
Short, cold	Increases	Increases	No change
Long, cold	Increases	Decreases (unless shivering occurs)	Decreases
Tepid	Increases	No change	Decreases
Long, hot	Decreases	Increases	Increases
Short, hot	Decreases	Increases	Increases
Very short, hot	Increases	Increases	Decreases

G. Principles of Fever Management

1. Fever can be beneficial.
2. Leave the fever alone (unless it is going to dangerous levels).
3. The patient should fast, slowly resuming eating when natural hunger returns.
4. Eating can resume when temperature is below 99.5 degrees F.
5. Sweating is good -- the body is working to maintain normal core temperature.
6. 102-103 degrees F (oral) is optimal for infection fighting.
7. Stop treatment before temperature reaches desired level, so you do not "overshoot" it.
8. "Long," cold treatments should last 10-30 minutes.
9. Always use friction with cold.
10. Always stop treatment if shivering occurs.
11. Neutral treatments should last from one to three hours.
12. Make certain the patient is well hydrated.

XII. HELIOTHERAPY

Heliotherapy is defined as the treatment of a patient by exposure to a form of light. The types of light commonly used in heliotherapy include: **Visible, Ultraviolet,** and **Infrared.** Discussed below are those most common forms of heliotherapy. Laser therapy is by definition a treatment with a form of light but is beyond the scope of this discussion.

The Electromagnetic Spectrum

ELF - Infra Sound - AM Radio - FM Radio - Microwaves - Infrared - ROYGBIV - Ultraviolet - X Ray - Gamma - Cosmic

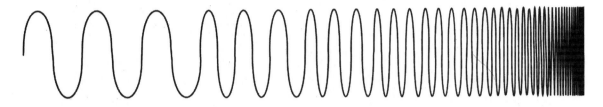

	Type	Wavelength	Frequency (Hz)	Use
Ionizing	Cosmic	.0001nm	3×10^{24}	
	Gamma	.01nm	3×10^{20}	Radium Therapy
	X-ray	50nm	3×10^{16}	Diagnostic & Therapy
	Ultraviolet	300nm	3×10^{15}	Dx, Tx, Vit D, Germicidal
Visible Light	Violet	390nm	$3\times10^{14+}$	
	Indigo			
	Blue			
	Green			Laser
	Yellow			(Including UV & IR)
	Orange			
	Red	770nm	3×10^{14}	
Near Infrared		770 - 1500 nm	300 GHz+	Radiant heating
Far Infrared		1500 - 12,500 nm		Radiant heating
Microwave		10-30nm	2450M	Heating
Shortwave		0.5-100mm	27M	Heating, Surgery
Television		10-30		
Radio		300	3K-3M	Music Therapy
Electric Power		5x1010	60	Muscle Stimulation
Extra Low Frequency		1,000-10,000km	30-300	"Qi Machine"

Electric (Visible) Light Bath

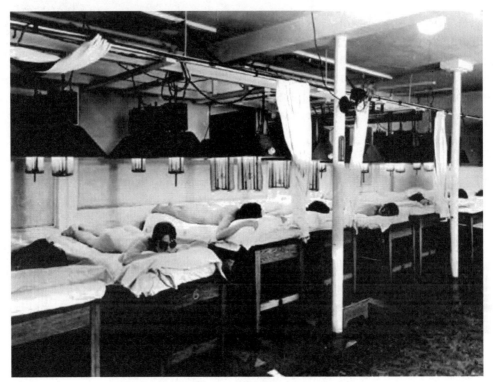

Electric Light Bath - Battlecreek Sanitarium - Circa 1925

- **Description:** An application of heat and light (full or partial spectrum) to the body by radiant energy, using incandescent light bulbs or laser.

- **Rationale:** Increased circulation and cellular metabolism result from the application of the radiant heat. Both muscular (visceral and skeletal) and connective tissues relax with heat.

- **Equipment:** Electric Light Cabinet or hand held lamp (for local application), Towels.

- **Procedure:** Patient sits in cabinet or is exposed to local light source for 10 to 30 minutes. Take care to avoid touching the light source. Protect sensitive body parts and have patient rest after treatment.

- **Indications:** Rheumatoid Arthritis, hypertension, muscular spasm/pain, decreased range of motion, prior to massage, and Seasonal Affective Disorder.

- **Contraindications:** Diabetes, peripheral vascular disease, cardiac impairment, inability to report, acute injury with inflammation, and with an emaciated patient.

Ultraviolet Light

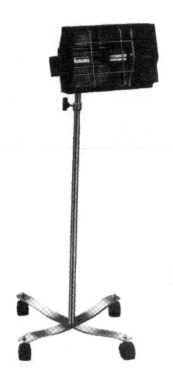

- **Description:** Application of ultraviolet light to the body. Ultraviolet light is defined as those frequencies between 180 and 400 nm and is produced when electrons of stable atoms move back and forth

- **Rationale:** Ultraviolet (UV) light rays are known to: be bactericidal, aid in the formation of Vit D, cause exfoliation of epidermal cells, increase production of red blood cells, thicken the epidermis, stimulate cellular metabolism, aid in wound healing, and stimulate the Pineal gland (thus decreasing the production of melatonin).

- **Equipment:** Commercial ultraviolet light lamp (hot or cold quartz) or sunlight. UV goggles and a watch with a second hand.

- **Procedure:** Place the UV source approximately 24 to 36 inches from the area to be treated (distance varies with type of device). Typical treatment time is 30 seconds for the first treatment, 60 seconds for the second and 90 seconds for each of the following treatments. With at least 24 hours between treatments,

> Doses of UV are described as: 1. "Suberythemal" (no redness), 2. "Minimal erythemal" (erythema lasting 24 hours), 3. "First - degree erythemal" (erythema lasting as long as 48 hours), 4. "Second-degree erythemal" (erythema with edema, peeling and pigmentation that lasts as long as 72 hours), 5. "Third-degree erythemal" (erythema with severe blistering and exudation and should be limited to an area less than 25 sq. cm.).

Cover eyes with UV goggles as well as body parts that are not going to be treated. Therapist should also use safety measures.

- **Indications:** Acne, Psoriasis, fungal and bacterial skin infections and Seasonal Affective Disorder

- **Contraindications:** Sensitivity to UV light, cancer, bleeding, Pellagra, Lupus, fever, active Tuberculosis and acute skin pathology. Some patients may have light sensitivity due to foods, medications, or disease. If in doubt, check with a physician.

Infrared Light

- **Description:**   Superficial heat treatment with the use of infrared light rays that are just beyond the red portion of visible light. Electromagnetic rays in the infrared light range are produced when a material is heated. Energy from the infrared light is transferred to tissue when the rays of light strike the skin. (Energy absorption, and thus heat production, is greatest when the light rays strike the body surface perpendicularly, at a 90 ° angle). The therapeutic and side- effects are similar to other local applications of heat.

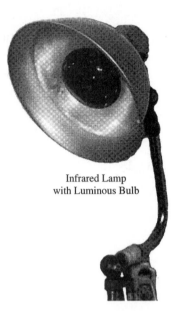

Infrared Lamp
with Luminous Bulb

- **Rationale:**   Increased circulation and cellular metabolism result from the application of local heat. Both muscular (visceral and skeletal) and connective tissues relax with heat.

- **Equipment:**   Commercial infrared lamp, goggles and towels. Two types of infrared devices are available, luminous and non-luminous. The luminous device produces rays with incandescent tungsten and carbide filament encased in a quartz tube and is similar to a light bulb. The non-luminous device often uses a metal coil, which radiates heat as electricity passes through it. Both types of units have a reflective hood that directs the radiation of heat in an even manner.

- **Procedure:**   Position lamp between 18 and 36 inches from body part being treated (distance varies with the type of lamp used), remove jewelry and protect sensitive body parts. Average treatment time is from 20 to 30 minutes. Have patient rest after treatment. * Increase distance if patient is uncomfortable or experiences more than slight or erythema. ** A moistened towel may be used to cover the treatment area - to create moist heating or to protect sensitive tissue (such as a decubitus ulcer).

- **Indications:**   Rheumatoid Arthritis, hypertension, muscular spasm/pain, decreased range of motion, and prior to massage.

- **Contraindications:** Diabetes, peripheral vascular disease, cardiac impairment, inability to report, acute injury w/ inflammation, and an emaciated patient.

Far Infrared Sauna - Hyperthermia

- **Description:** Full body exposure in an enclosed structure with Infrared heating unit(s). The ambient temperature is 100-130° F (compared to 180- 220° F in a traditional sauna)

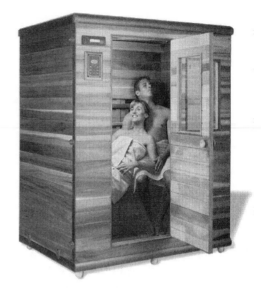

Far Infrared Sauna - Courtesy of Steam Embrace

- **Rationale*:** Infrared rays penetrate and heat tissues to a depth of 4 to 5 centimeters, thus stimulating cellular metabolism and peripheral circulation. Core body temperature may be raised to 101-102° F. Skeletal, smooth muscle and connective tissue relax with heat. Perspiration is increased (up to 500 grams per 30 minute session). Caloric expenditure is increased (600 to 800 calories per session). Sympathetic tone is decreased and a prolonged (at least 24 hour) vasodilation effect occurs. Lipophillic (organophosphate) toxins and heavy metals are excreted. Viruses are inactivated and the immune system stimulated.

- **Equipment:** Far-Infrared Sauna unit (available in hypoallergenic poplar wood)

- **Procedures:** Cleanse body with warm water (opens pores) before entering. Limit treatment time to 10-15 minutes, then increase to 25 or more minutes, as patient becomes "heat conditioned". Rest and cool-down. Drink plenty of fluids before and after treatment.

- **Indications:** Colds and flu; muscle spasms; joint stiffness; pain; weight control; and certain dermatological conditions. Detoxification and treatment of Hypertension, HIV and Cancer (by physicians orders).

- **Contraindications:** Patients with acute trauma, bleeding disorders, or who are pregnant. Those with Adrenal Dysfunction, MS, SLE, Cardiovascular Disease, Hypertension, Diabetes, PVD, Cancer, undiagnosed illness, or metal implants should consult their physician.

*A significant amount of current published research supports the above rationale.

Constitutional Treatment

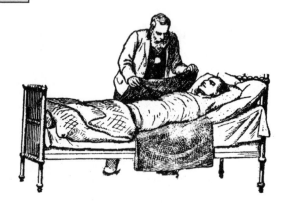

- **Description:**   This treatment was developed by Dr. O.G. Carroll and involves a series of alternating hot and cold applications to the chest, abdomen, and back while incorporating mild electrical stimulation (sine wave has traditionally been used) to the abdomen and back.

- **Rationale:**   Increased circulation and cellular metabolism, result from the application of alternate heat and cold. Muscular, connective, endocrine, vascular, and associated nervous tissues respond to both the thermal and electrical stimulation.

- **Equipment:**   Electrical stimulation unit, hot and cold water source, oral (or auricular) thermometer, hydrometer (for measuring the pre and post oral temperature and specific gravity of the patients urine). Pillow, 2 blankets, and at least 5 towels.

- **Procedure:**   Patient supine: place E-stim pads on back bilaterally at level of T_5, apply hot compress to chest and abdomen, and cover patient with blanket for duration of 5 minutes. Next: apply cold compress to chest and abdomen, and cover patient with blanket, apply E-stim (to patient tolerance) for duration of 10 minutes or until the compress begins to warm. Remove compresses, move E-stim pads to $T_{12} - L_1$ junction (over spinous processes), and to the abdomen at same level. Cover patient with blanket and apply E-stim to patient tolerance for duration of 10 minutes. Patient prone: repeat contrast compresses to back (5 and 10 min. respectively without E-stim). Have patient rest, record data, and schedule next treatment.

- **Indications:**   Digestive, endocrine, dermatological, circulatory and respiratory complaints, infectious diseases and immune deficiencies, PMS, arthritis, mood disorders, and obesity.

- **Contraindications:** Acute cystitis, acute asthma, a chilled patient, pregnancy, and the standard contraindications for electrical stimulation.

Glossary

Ablution:	Applying water by hand to wash or cleanse. The hand is covered with a bath mitt or towel (or water is poured over the body).
Acidosis:	An excessive acidity of body fluids due to an accumulation of acids, or a loss of bicarbonate. The hydrogen ion concentration is increased, thus the pH is decreased.
Acute:	Having rapid onset, severe symptoms, and short duration. Opposite of chronic.
Afferent:	Conveying a nerve impulse (or liquid) toward an organ or area.
Affusion:	A stream of water is poured on the body with the intention of lowering a fever by lowering the body temperature.
Alternate:	Contrasting hot and cold applications to a body area. These applications consist of at least three applications of cold and hot. The cold application is 1/4 to 1/2 as long as the duration of the heat application, beginning with heat and ending with cold.
Analgesic:	Relieving pain without affecting consciousness.
Anesthetic:	A substance or reaction that reduces pain.
Anion:	A negatively charged ion such as Cl^- or O^{2-}.
Anodyne:	An agent for pain reduction.
Antipyretic:	An agent used in reduction of fever.
Antispasmodic:	An agent which reduces spasms.
Arteriosclerosis:	(Atherosclerosis) - Term applied to a variety of conditions where there is thickening, hardening, and/or loss of elasticity of the artery walls, resulting in altered function of tissues and organs.
Axon:	Long cytoplasmic process of a neuron (nerve cell).
Balneology:	The branch of science concerned with mineral waters and their therapeutic uses, especially as a bath.
Balneotherapy:	The application of mineral waters for therapeutic purposes.
Baroreceptor:	A sense organ (nerve terminal) that responds to changes in pressure.
Bradykinin:	A potent vasodilator (inflammatory) polypeptide hormone.
Calorie:	The same as specific heat, the standard of thermic measure which is the amount of heat required to raise one gram of water one degree Celsius at sea level.
Cation:	A positively charged ion such as Na^+ or Mg^{2+}.
Chemotaxis:	The ability of white blood cells to locate and attack pathogens.
Chronic:	A disease or illness of long duration and showing little change. Opposite of acute.
Circadian Rhythm:	Pertains to events that occur at approximately 24-hour intervals, such as certain physiological phenomena.
Clyster:	An enema - fluid ejection into the rectum.
Collagen:	Supportive protein component of connective tissue, bone, cartilage, and skin which will convert into gelatin when boiled.

196

Concentration:	A measure of the quantity of solutes dissolved in a specified amount of solute.
Compress:	A moist, folded pad of material (possibly medicated) applied with pressure.
Constitutional Treatment:	Developed by Dr. Harold Dick, includes a series of hot and cold compresses applied to the chest and back, in conjunction with mild electrical stimulation (Sine wave) to the back and abdomen.
Colloidal Particles:	Solute particles that are very large (1-100nm) in solution, they may be proteins, or aggregates of molecules, atoms, or electrolytes
Colloids:	Solutions containing colloidal particles.
Crenology (Crenotherapy):	The therapeutic use of water from mineral springs.
Cryotherapy:	The therapeutic use of local cold applications.
Dendrite:	One of the cytoplasmic branches of nerve cells (neurons), which conducts the impulses received from the termination of other neurons toward the cell body.
Depletion:	The result of derivation--reducing the amount of blood in a congested area by increasing it in another body part, usually by cold applications.
Depressant:	Similar to a sedative in which the various vital activities are decreased.
Dermatome:	The skin area supplied by the sensory fibers of a single spinal nerve.
Derivation:	Drawing blood or lymph *from* one body part by increasing the amount in *another* body part (local affect of heat).
Diapedesis:	Movement of cells into circulation.
Diaphoretic:	To increase sweating.
Diuresis:	The act of increasing the production of urine.
Diurnal:	Occurring during the day.
Douche:	A stream of water directed against a part of the body or into a body cavity.
Edema:	Retention of excessive amounts of fluid by the body tissues.
Efferent:	Conveying a nerve impulse (or liquid) away from an organ or area.
Elastin:	A yellow scleroprotein present in elastic fibers that allows them to stretch about 1 and 1/2 times their original length.
Electrolytes:	Ionized salts in blood, tissue fluids, and cells including salts of sodium, chloride, and potassium.
Enzymes:	Any one of the numerous complex proteins that are produced by living cells, which catalyze accelerate, and promote specific biochemical reactions.
Erythema:	Redness of the skin.
Excitant:	That which increases the activity of a function.
Febrile:	Pertaining to a fever, feverish.

197

Fluxion:	Active or arterial hyperemia--a great increase in the rapidity of the blood current in a particular body part.
Fomentation:	A very *hot*, moist application (frequently made of wool), which can be medicated.
Ganglion:	A collection of nerve cell bodies located outside the brain or spinal cord.
Heating Compress:	A *cold* compress, usually covered by dry flannel, which is applied to a body part. This compress becomes heated by the body because of the increased circulation. The cold compress stimulates the local area.
Histamine:	A white crystalline amine, when released within the body, causes bronchiolar constriction, arteriolar dilatation, increased gastric secretion, and a fall in blood pressure.
Homeostasis:	A state of physiologic equilibrium in the living body under variations in the environment.
Hyperthermia:	Extremely high body temperature.
Hypertonic:	A solution that has a higher osmotic pressure (greater solute concentration) than the cells of the body.
Hypotonic:	A solution that has a lower osmotic pressure (lower solute concentration) than the cells of the body.
Hydrochloric Acid:	A colorless compound of hydrogen chloride (HCl) and the acid secreted by the stomach.
Hydrostatic:	Relating to the pressure exerted by liquids at rest.
Hypnotic:	Something that induces sleep.
Hypodermis:	Subcutaneous fascia.
Inflammation:	A condition in which there is redness, heat, swelling, and pain. It may be caused by an infection, bruising, chemical irritation, or strain of a body part.
Interleukin-1:	A polypeptide with fever-inducing and lymphocyte-activating properties.
Intrinsic:	It is the direct result of an action.
Ion:	An atom with an electrical charge because of having a different number of protons and electrons.
Ischemia:	Lack of blood in an area of the body due to mechanical obstruction or functional constriction of a blood vessel.
Latent Heat:	The extra calories given off when freezing water is being lowered 1 degree C. Approximately 80 calories of heat must be lost before water can change its state from liquid to solid. Stated another way, when ice melts to a liquid state, it requires the energy stored in the water.
Lesion:	A morbid change in the structure or function of tissues, due to injury or disease.
Leukocytosis:	Abnormal increase in the number of white corpuscles in the blood.
Macrophage:	A large mononuclear cell which ingests degenerated cells and blood tissue.

Mask: (**Masque**)	A skin treatment where the fruit, mud, seaweed, herbs, or paraffin is left on the skin of the face or body for an extended period of time to; cleanse, dry, moisturize, exfoliate, or soothe.
Mechanoreceptors:	A receptor that responds to the stimulation of mechanical pressure.
Motility:	Ability to move spontaneously.
Motor:	Producing movement by conveying impulses form nerve centers to the muscle.
Necrosis:	Death of cells or tissue within a circumscribed area.
Neuron:	A nerve cell capable of carrying an impulse.
Nociceptor:	Peripheral nerve organ that receives and transmits painful sensations.
Osmosis:	The movement of water through a semi-permeable membrane from an area of high concentration to one of low concentration.
Osmotic pressure:	The pressure created by a dissolved substance that cannot pass through a semi permeable membrane.
Pathogens:	A micro-organism or substance capable of causing disease.
pH level:	The degree of alkalinity or acidity of a solution.
Piloerection:	Erection of hairs.
Pyrogen:	A fever producing agent.
Poultice: (**Cataplasm**)	A soft, moist, hot mass spread between a layered cloth, applied to a given body area. The intent is to create moist, local heat, or counterirritation.
Prostaglandin:	A hormone-like substance produced and exerting its influence in localized tissues.
Purgative:	Substance causing vomiting or bowel evacuation.
Reflex:	An involuntary and immediate response to a stimulus that occurs in various body structures.
Retrostasis:	Driving blood/lymph *from* one body area *to* another (internal organs).
Revulsion:	Single, prolonged application of heat followed by a single brief application of cold (movement of blood out of an area-- local affects of cold).
Sensory:	Relating to sensation.
Serotonin:	A neurotransmitter responsible for smooth muscle contraction.
Solute:	The component in a solution that changes it's state upon dissolving.
Solution:	A uniform mixture of two or more components.
Solvent:	The dissolving material in a solution, the component whose state does not change
Somatic:	Pertaining to the body.
Sphincter:	Any circular muscle that, when contracted, closes a natural body opening.
Specific Heat:	The number of calories required to raise the temperature of one gram of a substance one degree centigrade. Every substance has its own specific heat.
Stimulant:	Increases nerve activity.

Sudoriferous:	Producing or carrying perspiration.
Sudoresis:	Same as diaphoresis - profuse sweating.
Suspension:	A mixture in which the particles are so large that they settle out.
Synapse:	The site of communication between two nerve cells.
Tetanic:	Intermittent muscle spasm, usually beginning with sharp flexion of the wrists and ankles, but can involve other muscles. Consists of at least 30 individual contractions per second.
Tonic:	A remedy that increases vigor (such as a cold shower).
Vascular shunting:	Bypassing or diverting blood flow in the vessels.
Vasoconstriction:	Narrowing of the lumen of blood vessels, especially arterioles.
Vasodilatation:	The increase in the diameter of blood vessels or lymph vessels.
Vasomotor:	Pertaining to the motion of the blood vessels.
Visceral:	Pertaining to internal organs.
Viscoelastic:	The flexible nature of a substance which is dependent upon its degree of molecular cohesion.
Viscosity:	The degree of resistance to the flow of a substance.

NOTES

The grand show is eternal ......on seas and continents and islands – John Muir

WORKS CITED:

Anderson, Debi, *The Transition to Day Spas*, Skin Inc.--September/October, 1995.

Bates and Hanson, *Aquatic Exercise Therapy*, W.B. Saunders Co. Philadelphia, PA, 1996.

Boyle, Wade, N.D. and Saine, Andre', N.D., *Lectures in Naturopathic Hydrotherapy*, Buckeye Naturopathic Press, East Palestine, OH, 1988.

Bergel, Dr. Reinhard R., Ph.D. & Director, H.E.A.T. *Spa Therapy Training--Spa Practices & Operations* and *Hydro & Herbal Therapy--The Kneipp System*, Calistoga, CA, 94515.

Bergel, Dr. Reinhard R., Ph.D., *Balneotherapy--The Systematic Application of Mineral Water for Therapeutic Purposes*, Massage & Bodywork Quarterly – Fall, 1994.

Brown, Monica T., *Evolution & Essence of Spa Therapies*, Massage & Bodywork—Summer, 1995.

Burton-Goldberg Group, *Alternative Medicine-the Definitive Guide*, Future Medicine Publishing Inc., Puyallup, WA, 1993.

Cailliet, Rene, M.D., *Pain Mechanisms and Management*, F. A Davis Co., Philadelphia, PA, 1993.

Cameron, Michelle H., *Physical Agents In Rehabilitation*, W.B. Saunders Co, Philadelphia, PA, 1999.

Carbone, David James, L.M.T., *The Power of Paraffin*, Body Therapy--November/December, 1993.

Croutier, Alev Lytle, *Taking the Waters--Spirit-Art-Sensuality*, Abbeville Press: New York, NY, 1992.

Dail, and Thomas, *Hydrotherapy – Simple Treatment for Common Ailments*, Teach Services Inc, Brushton, NY, 1995.

De Vierville, J. Paul Ph.D., *Taking the Waters*, Massage & Bodywork – February, 2000.

Deiss, Joseph Jay, *Herculaneum, Italy's Buried Treasure*, Harper & Row, Publishers, NY, NY, 1985.

Dox, Ida G., Ph.D., Melloni, B. John, Ph.D., and Eisner, Gilbert M., M.D. *The Harper Collins Illustrated Medical Dictionary*, Harper Perennial Publishers, NY, NY, 1993.

Fox, Stuart I., *Human Physiology,* Wm. C. Brown Publishers, Dubuque, IA, 1993.

Friel, John P., *Dorland's Illustrated Medical Dictionary*, W. B. Saunders Co., United States, 1974.

Mosby's Medical Nursing and Allied Health Dictionary, Harcourt Health Sciences Inc. St. Louis, MO, 2002.

Guyton, Arthur C. and Hall, John E., *Textbook of Medical Physiology*, W.B. Saunders Co, Philadelphia, PA, 1996.

Hecox, Bernadette; Mehreteab, Tsega A; and Weisberg, Joseph, *Physical Agents, A Comprehensive Text for Physical Therapists*, Appleton & Lange, Norwalk, CT, 1994.

Hole, John W. Jr., *Essentials of Human Anatomy & Physiology*, Wm. C. Brown Publishers, Dubuque, IA, 1992.

Holmes, Peter, L.Ac., M.H., *Aromatherapy--Applications for Clinical Practice*, Alternative & Complementary Therapies--April/May, 1995.

Johnson, A.C., D.C., *Chiropractic Drugless Therapy*, Self-Published, 1965.

Kahn, Joseph, *Principles and Practice of Electrotherapy*, 4th Edition, Churchill Livingstone, New York, NY, 2000.

Kellogg, J.H., M.D., *Rational Hydrotherapy*, Modern Medicine Pub. Co., Battle Creek, MI, 1923.

Lehmann, Justus F., *Therapeutic Heat and Cold*, Williams & Wilkins, Baltimore, MD, 1990.

LeRoy, B.R., M.A., M.D., and LeRoy, B.R. Jr., A.B., *Practical Colonic Irrigation*, Spartan Press, Seattle, WA, 1933.

Lindlahr, Victor H., *The Natural Way to Health*, Newcastle Publishing Co. Inc., 1973.

Moor, Fred B., Peterson, Stella C., Manwell, Ethel M., Noble, Mary C. and Muench, Gertrude, *Manual of Hydrotherapy and Massage*, Pacific Press Publishing Association, Mountain View, CA, 1964.

Murray, Michael and Pizzorno, Joseph, N.D., *Encyclopedia of Natural Medicine*, Prima Publishing, Rocklin, CA, 1991.

Myers, Rose Sgarlat, *Saunders Manual of Physical Therapy Practice*, W.B. Saunders Co, Philadelphia, PA, 1995.

Nikola, R.J., L.M.T., *Creatures of Water*, Europa Therapeutic, Salt Lake City, UT, 1995.

Raney, Marian S., *Hydrating Body Treatment with Paraffin--How To*, Skin Inc., September/October, 1994.

Raney, Marian S., *Purifying Body Mask--How To*, Skin Inc., September/October, 1995.

Ryrie, Charlie, *The Healing Energies of Water*, Journey Editions, Boston, MA, 1999.

Shankar and Randall, *Therapeutic Physical Modalities*, Hanley & Belfus Inc., Medical Publishers, Philadelphia, PA, 2002.

Thibodeau and Patton, *The Human Body in Health and Disease*, Mosby Year Book, St. Louis, MO, 1992.

Thrash, Agatha and Calvin, MDs, *Home Remedies*, Thrash Publications, Seale, AL, 1981.

Tortora and Grabowski, *Principles of Anatomy and Physiology*, 10th Edition, John Wiley & Sons, New York, NY, 2003.

Trivieri and Anderson, *Alternative Medicine, the Definitive Guide*, Celestial Arts, Berkeley, CA, 2002.

Warwick, Robert, and Williams, Peter, *Gray's Anatomy*, W. B. Saunders Co., Philadelphia, PA, 2000.

Wendel, Dr. Paul, *Father Kneipp's Health Teachings*, Published by Dr. Paul Wendel, Brooklyn, NY, 1947.

Water

Water, sculptor of earth, refreshing, giver of life.

Endlessly changing color and hue, light in refraction mirrors a world in continual change.

It cleanses the earth.

Weaver of stories, the power of the sky revealed in the rain.

To dive into it is to search for the ultimate mystery.

Honor it.

(Author unknown)

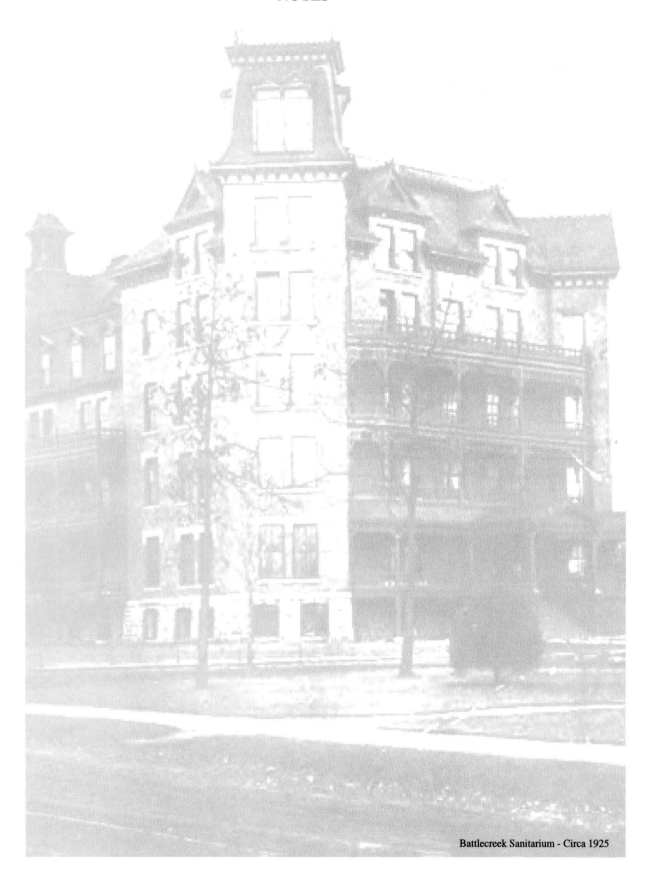

Battlecreek Sanitarium - Circa 1925

RESOURCE DIRECTORY:

Alar Flotation Systems
Joseph Baker, Manager
10100 International Drive
Orlando, FL 32821
Tel: 407-352-7741
Fax: 407-351-0690
Manufactures & suppliers of sensory deprivation (floatation) tanks.

American Spa Therapy Education & Certification Council (ASTECC)
1014 N. Olive St.
West Palm Beach, FL 33401
Tel: 561-802-3855
Fax: 561-802-6642
Website: www.bramhamspa.com
Non-profit organization dedicated to maintaining standards of quality for education of
spa professionals.

AMI inc. (Aqua PT)
P.O. Box 808
Groton, CT 06340
Tel: 860-536-3735
Fax: 860-536-4362
Website: www.aquapt.com
Manufactures & suppliers of Aqua PT dry hydrotherapy – massage device.

Aquatics Resources Network
Andrea Salzman, PT
302 160th St, Suite 200
Amery, WI 54001
Tel: 715-248-7258
Fax: 715-248-3065
Website: www.aquaticnet.com
Professional Association fostering appropriate use of aquatic therapy through
communication, education, and research. Publishes monthly newsletter.

Bramham Institute & Spa
Anne Bramham, President
1014 N. Olive St.
West Palm Beach, FL 33401
Tel: 561-802-3855
Fax: 561-802-6642
Website: www.bramhamspa.com
Providers of on-site training and certification in Spa Therapy and Spa Management.

Chattanooga Group Inc.
PO Box 489
Hixson, TN 37343
Tel: 800-592-2281
Website: www.chattgroup.com
Suppliers of the "Hydrocollator" moist heat therapy device.

Corso Enterprises Inc.
Cryo-Therapy Division
1001 Bridgeway, Suite 449
Sausalito, CA 94965
Tel: 415-332-4607
Fax: 415-332-1621
Website: www.eyespack.com
Manufacturers and suppliers of cryotherapy & heat therapy compresses.

Cosmopro Inc. & Pevonia International
Philippe Hennessy, President
284 Fentress Blvd.
Daytona Beach, FL
Tel: 386-239-8972
Fax: 386-239-8269
Website: www.cosmopro.com & www.pevonia.com
Manufactures and suppliers of hydrotherapy & spa equipment and products.

H.E.A.T.
Reinhard R. Bergel, Ph. D.
P.O. Box 1177
Calistoga, CA 94515
Tel: 800-473-4328
Fax: 707-942-0734
Supplier of hydrotherapy & spa equipment, products, and training.

Health Research Books
PO Box 850
Pomeroy, WA 99347
Tel: 888-844-2386
Fax: 509-843-2387
Website: www.healthresearchbooks.com
Publisher & supplier of hydrotherapy and other health related books.

Himalayan Institute Press
RR 1 Box 405
Honesdale, PA 18431
Tel: 800-822-4547
Fax: 570-253-6360
Website: www.himalayaninstitute.org
Suppliers of the Neti Pot (nasal irrigation device), Ayurvedic products, books, tapes, classes, seminars, and health care services.

International Association for Colon Hydrotherapy
PO Box 461285
San Antonio, TX 78246
Tel: 210-366-2888
Fax: 210-366-2999
Website: www.i-act.org
Association supporting educational standards and professionalism in colon therapy.

International Clinical Hyperthermia Society
Homayoon Shidnia, M.D.
1502 East County Line Rd.
Indianapolis, IN 46227
Tel: 317-887-7651
Fax: 21317-887-7650
Website: www.hyperthermia-ichs.org
Society supporting educational standards and professionalism in hyperthermia.

International Society of Medical Hydrology & Climatology
Torpin 13
D-17111 Sarow / Germany
Website: www.ismh.web
Professional association dedicated to the design, planning, and coordination of research in the field of Health Resort Medicine and Spa Therapy.

International Spa Association
2365 Harrodsburg Rd., Ste A-325
Lexington, KY 40504
Tel: 859-226-4372
Website: www.experienceispa.com
Professional association supporting spa education, standard setting, and resource sharing.

Jonathan Paul DeVierville, PhD
c/o Alamo Plaza Spa
226 Woodcrest Dr.
San Antonio, TX 78209
Tel: 210-822-7238
Website: www.alamoplazaspa.com
Director of "Kur Spa Course" at the Karlsbad Spa in the Czech Republic.

Kneipp Corporation of America
Attn: Joella Bury
105-107 Stonehurst Court
Northvale, NJ 07647
Tel: 800-937-4372
Fax: 201-750-2070
Importers and distributors of Kneipp products.

Liquid Sound
Attn: Marion Schneider
Klinikzentrum Bad Sulza
Ruldolf-Groschner str. 11
D-99518 Bad Sulza, Germany
Tel: + 49 (0) 36461-90
Website: www.kbs.de
Developers of Liquid Sound Therapy at Bad Sulza, Germany.

Orthocare
18011 Mitchell South
Irvine, CA 92614
Tel: 800-266-6969
Fax: 800-821-8012
Orthopedic Surgical and Rehabilitation Products
Manufactures & distributors of self-refrigerating cold packs and splints.

Samadhi Tank Co. Inc.
2123 Lake Shore Ave.
Los Angeles, CA 90039
Tel: 210-822-7238
Manufactures & distributors of Samadhi sensory deprivation (float) tanks.

Sterling Institute
Marian Urban
513 Camino De Los Marquez
Sante Fe, NM 87501
Tel: 505-984-3223
Fax: 505-988-5644
Traditional Kneipp spa therapy training.

T.H. Stone, LLC
Sonia Alexandra
4521 North Dixie Hwy
Boca Raton, FL 33431
Tel: 866-680-5149
Fax: 561-361-3965
Website: www.thstone.com   Suppliers of stone therapy equipment and training.

Thalasso Systems & Hydro Spa Consulting
Philippe Therene, President
PO Box 1093
Calistoga, CA 94515
Tel: 707-942-5198
Fax: 707-942-6198
Website: www.thalassosystems.com & www.hydrospaconsulting.com
Manufactures and suppliers of hydrotherapy & spa equipment and products.
Spa facility design and development.

Therabath
WR Medical Electronics Co.
123 North Second Street
Stillwater, MN 55082
Tel: 800-321-6387
Fax: 651-439-9733
Website: www.therabathpro.com
Manufactures and suppliers of professional paraffin baths.

Touch America
PO Box 1304
Hillsborough, NC 27278
Tel: 800-678-6824
Fax: 919- 732-1173
Website: www.touchamerica.com
Manufactures and suppliers of hydrotherapy & spa equipment and training.

Watsu Oasis
Tal Hurley, CMT
Desert Hot Springs, CA
Tel: 760-329-1214
Website: www.watsuoasis.com
Professional Watsu educator and practitioner.

Worldwide Aquatic Bodywork Association (W.A.B.A.)
PO Box 889
Middletown, CA 95461
Tel: 707-987-3801
Fax: 707-987-9638
Website: www.waba.edu
Professional association supporting education & resource sharing regarding Watsu and
Aquatic Bodywork.

INDEX

NOTES

"Water Is the Blue Soul of the Planet" - *Dr. Pedro Arrojo Agundo*